Health & Wellness

Secrets
That Will
Change
Your
Life

Mark A. Finley and Peter N. Landless, Editors

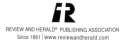

REVIEW AND HERALD® PUBLISHING ASSOCIATION
Since 1861 | www.reviewandherald.com

The Review and Herald® Publishing Association publishes biblically based materials for spiritual, physical, and mental growth and Christian discipleship.

Unless otherwise noted, Bible texts in this book are from the King James Version.

Scripture quotations credited to NIV are from the *Holy Bible , New International Version.* Copyright © 1973, 1978, 1984, 2011 by Biblica, Inc. Used by permission. All rights reserved worldwide.

Texts credited to NKJV are from the New King James Version. Copyright © 1979, 1980, 1982 by Thomas Nelson, Inc. Used by permission. All rights reserved.

Edited by Gerald Wheeler
Copyedited by Jeremy J. Johnson and Ted Hessel
Interior design by Emily Ford/Review and Herald Design Center
Cover design by Bryan Gray/Review and Herald Design Center
Cover art © Thinkstock

PRINTED IN U.S.A.
18 17 16 15 14   5 4 3 2 1

Library of Congress Control Number: 2014936041

ISBN 978-0-8280-2803-5

CONTENTS

Preface

Why You Need This Book

Healthy choices lead to healthier lives: choose to live.

A list of the 100 confirmed oldest people in modern times in the world ranges from 113 to 122 years.[1] Only six of these supercentenarians were still alive at the beginning of 2014, but many others can appear in the future. Medicine promises to increase considerably human life expectancy during the next decades. Until then, you can do your own part to live longer and better. While research on twins suggests that 20 to 30 percent of a person's life span is related to genetics, many other studies have shown that longevity depends greatly on lifestyle.[2]

Modern medicine has created sophisticated techniques to improve human health. Yet nobody who knows the figures can say that the war has been won. Seeking health is a daily challenge for every government and each person. If you like numbers, here are a few facts:

- The estimated global health-care services market for 2015 is $3 trillion, which makes the health-care industry one of the largest sectors of the world economy. In most developed countries health care consumes more than 10 percent of the gross domestic product.
- The global pharmaceuticals market is worth more than $300 billion a year. The 10 largest drug companies (six based in the United States and four in Europe) have sales of more than $10 billion a year and profit margins of about 30 percent. On the other hand, the cost to develop a single drug may surpass $1.3 billion.[3]
- Worldwide, according to the World Health Organization, in 2006 there were more than 59 million health workers, including 9.2 million physicians, 19.4 million nurses and midwives, 1.9 million dentists and other dentistry personnel, 2.6 million pharmacists and other pharmaceutical personnel, and more than 1.3 million community health staffers. Those numbers would be

even larger today. However, even then there was a shortage of more than 4 million physicians, nurses, midwives, and others.[4]

- Unnecessary suffering is still a grave problem in the world, for only one in 10 of those who need palliative care, including pain relief, currently receive it.[5]

- Just in the United States alone, according to a study from Georgetown University's Center on Education and the Workforce, it is estimated that the health industry must create 5.6 million new jobs by 2020 to meet the growing demand.[6]

- One big challenge today is the aging of society. The global population is getting older. It has been predicted that by 2050 the percentage of people more than 60 years of age will increase from 21 percent today to 32 percent in developed countries and from 8 percent to 20 percent in less-developed nations.[7]

Health is the dream of poor and rich alike. "When I was an intern at Johns Hopkins," Dr. Ben Carson, a famous neurosurgeon, reports, "I was very impressed by the caliber of patients that I saw on the wards. There were many heads of state, royalty, and heads of many large organizations. Many of them were dying of horrible diseases and would gladly have given every title and every penny for a clean bill of health. This really puts into perspective the things that are truly important in life."

In fact, without health most other things are not that important. For this reason we need to pay a great deal of attention to the maintenance of good health and not just become concerned when something threatens it. And when we talk about health, we must think not only of its physical dimension, but also of its mental and spiritual facets. Our duty is to optimize all three of these aspects in our own lives and in the lives of everyone else in the world. "As a physician, I have frequently been able to witness the joy associated with restored physical and emotional health," Dr. Carson reveals, "but this is minor compared to the potentially everlasting joy associated with spiritual health."

The world has become such a complex, dangerous, and sick place that making good choices is more important than ever. To minimize or prevent problems is the best strategy to have a safer and more fulfilling life. Here enters the message of this book, whose aim is to help people improve their quality of life.

Most likely you have begun reading this book because you desire to live a longer, healthier, and happier life. That is a noble goal, because you have been made to live forever. If you follow the principles and tips presented here, this dream may come true. You deserve to live well and be happy.

Furthermore, we are much more valuable than may appear at a casual glance. Take the human body, for example. When researchers add up the chemical value of our body's component parts, they might conclude that we are not worth much. Yet even then *Wired* magazine estimates that if we consider the monetary value of our hearts, lungs, kidneys, DNA, and bone marrow, we are individually worth up to a whopping $45 million.

As a rational, thinking, living human being with the enormous capacity to love and experience life's greatest joys, you are even more valuable than $45 million, and that is what this book is all about. You are embarking on a journey of discovery that has the potential to be life-changing. The principles of better living and the practical lifestyle suggestions you will discover in every chapter can make a real difference in the quality of your life. You can live life to the fullest and discover joy to the max.

As you scan these pages and consider your personal health, you will recognize that to achieve life's greatest happiness you will probably need to make some positive steps. But rather than overwhelming yourself with multiple changes, choose to begin by taking a few small steps at first. For example, as you succeed in increasing your exercise, or reducing the amount of sugar and refined foods in your diet or getting more rest, your resolve will increase, and your ability to make healthy choices will become stronger.

Good health is a state that we all desire, but sadly, many people realize its worth and value only once they've lost it! Here is an opportunity for you to evaluate your health and lifestyle carefully, not just hastily make a few resolutions that rapidly fly out the window. Do you feel that you're getting the best out of life in all its facets? Have you recently assessed your *total* health, including its physical, mental, social, and spiritual aspects?

You may assume that you manage your day-to-day routines of

eating, working, and sleeping quite well. But are you enjoying a real quality of life? Have you ever considered that life may have much more to it than you are currently experiencing?

Medical Progress

During the twentieth century medical science made great strides toward increased good health as its understanding of physiology and disease processes grew. Public health measures that improved sanitation, sewage disposal, and the delivery of clean water to communities positively affected both the quality and longevity of life for millions. The development of vaccinations and immunizations—one of the most cost-effective ways of preventing infectious diseases—eradicated smallpox toward the end of the twentieth century and greatly decreased the ravages of polio and diphtheria. Reported cases of measles, mumps, rubella, tetanus, and diphtheria have plummeted about 90 percent because of immunizations.

Infectious and communicable diseases—those spread by bacteria, viruses, fungi, and parasites (for example, tuberculosis, malaria, and hepatitis)—continue to cause significant problems worldwide. And HIV and AIDS claimed the lives of an estimated 1.7 million people in 2011 alone. Yet we cannot underestimate the tremendous strides in health care.

Unfortunately, such advances in medicine also have another side to them. As world governments and public health experts focused on treating, controlling, or eliminating infectious (or communicable) diseases, noncommunicable or lifestyle ones skyrocketed. Today such noncommunicable diseases have become entrenched in all societies of the world—developed and emerging economies, affluent and poor. They are mainly lifestyle-related and pose a huge threat to our health, happiness, and longevity. It is highly likely that someone close to you has died because of cancer, coronary heart disease, stroke, diabetes, or chronic respiratory diseases.

What Is *Your* Health Issue?

You may be feeling good up to now because you do not smoke tobacco or drink alcohol, but what about your diet and salt intake?

The foods we choose to eat largely produce the various noncommunicable diseases. At least 40 percent of all deaths from these kinds of diseases result from the consumption of foods high in saturated and trans fats, salt, and sugar (and refined carbohydrates). Are you selecting your foods wisely and carefully, focusing on variety and good nutrition within the bounds of your budget? Simple actions such as cutting back on salt, reducing food portion sizes, and eating more fruits and vegetables can make a huge difference to your health. If you are into junk foods, irregular meals, excessive salt, large amounts of fat, a highly refined food diet, or large portions, know that life can be much better, and that's why this book is just for you.

Of course, to enjoy the best health possible you should be exercising daily. You might say, "I get up off the couch for a snack during every TV commercial, and I walk the 100 feet from the closest parking spot to the grocery store." But do you have a regularly planned, systematic exercise program?

Health professionals encourage us to walk 10,000 steps daily! We should be physically active for at least 30 minutes each day in order for our wonderful body to function at its best. So if you're groaning that you're too busy to exercise, but really want to begin a practical, sustainable exercise program, keep reading.

What about your interpersonal relationships? Do you have friends you care about, younger people you mentor, individuals in need whom you help? Social support and connectedness to God and others are also health-giving! Perhaps you have broken relationships in your life that need mending. Keep reading. God has a plan for you that is far better than you can ever imagine.

Are you happy? Do you wake up with purpose, walk with "pep in your step," and have a smile on your face? Or has life become too much? Are you anxious or downhearted? Does the future look bleak? Do you struggle with dark thoughts of meaninglessness, failure, and defeat? As we explore scientific facts and discover life-changing principles of the Bible that we can universally apply, you will see that the possibility of happiness is real.

We can almost guarantee that disappointment, heartache, and trials will afflict our lives at times, because we dwell in a sin-filled world. But God is bigger than our trials, greater than our difficulties, and larger than our challenges. We may be weak, but He is strong. God is our assurance when we face uncertainty. Should guilt threaten to overwhelm us, He can be our peace. He is our wisdom when we find ourselves perplexed. When we are imprisoned in the chains of seemingly unbreakable habits, He stands ready to offer supernatural power to free us. And when we are lonely, He is forever near.

Thus, whenever we face paralyzing anxiety and overwhelming fear, God's words still speak to our hearts: "Come to Me, all you who labor and are heavy laden, and I will give you rest" (Matthew 11:28, NKJV). Should the burdens of life appear insurmountable, He urges us to cast "all of our care upon Him, for He cares" for us (1 Peter 5:7, NKJV). And when the future seems uncertain, He reminds us: "Fear not for I am with you; be not dismayed for I am your God. I will strengthen you. Yes, I will help you, I will uphold you with My righteous right hand" (Isaiah 41:10, NKJV).

In God we will find rest and hope for the future. Our loving heavenly Father has given us a road map and instructions on how to have health and wellness—now and beyond, and even into eternity! We were born for something much more than just struggling through a few decades and then dying. God intended for us to live the abundant life today, tomorrow, and forever.

The Lord has a plan for your life that is far more than amazing. As His personal concern, He wants you to live life in all of its fullness. He longs that you experience joy beyond measure. In fact, Jesus said: "I have come that they may have life, and that they may have it more abundantly" (John 10:10, NKJV). Heaven's plan for you is a life of physical, mental, emotional, and spiritual wholeness.

Each chapter in this book is an adventure into really living. As you put their principles into practice, you will notice positive changes in your life. Some of the benefits of your healthful choices will be almost immediate, but most of them will come gradually. Don't become discouraged or give up too quickly. Continue to make positive lifestyle choices, and in time you will be astounded with what is happening in your life.

A loving God made us with the power of choice. Our wills, the governing power deep within our nature that enables us to choose the way we think, the physical habits we develop, and the spiritual decisions we make, are a powerful force in lifestyle transformation. Current medical research is leaning more and more in the direction that, although our genetics do play a role in determining the state of our well-being and overall health, choice is a much more influential and important factor. Our health is not simply a matter of chance. It has a great deal to do with our daily decisions.

When we choose to make positive choices, the Holy Spirit comes to our aid to enable us to put those decisions into practice. All of heaven's power is available to us. Your will may be weakened because of poor choices, but it is never too late to begin to make healthy ones. You can take charge of your life and health. Change always begins with choice, and it occurs when we realize we are not mere victims of chance, but have the freedom to take responsibility for our own health and happiness. Those who decide to adopt the suggestions given here will undoubtedly experience a fuller quality and enjoyment of life.

Of course, self-improvement has its limitations. Our biological realities remind us of some insurmountable barriers and define the extent of human accomplishment. But the beauty and value of this book is that it offers more than is humanly attainable. As you read it, you will inevitably realize that you can rely on a gracious higher power. The experience of a spirituality born of a relationship with a loving God can make a huge difference in your life.

While we are finite, God and His grace are infinite. Grace is the power of the omnipotent to grant to the impotent the ability to be whole—all accomplished through the construction of a relationship. As we focus on the whole person—physical, mental, and spiritual—God offers us life full of health and wellness. He rains grace down upon us from heaven, traversing a gulf that we cannot possibly span. Given to the undeserving in incomprehensible love, grace permits the experience of a full and abundant life not only here and now, but also for eternity.

In our earthly life, despite our best efforts and compliance with healthful principles, we cannot escape the lingering shadow of our mortality. But when a human being reaches across the gap between us and God, hope is born! Love rattles the bars of the dungeons of death. Graves will yet yield to the persuasion of grace. If you desire to improve your health, science can help you. But if you want to live forever, seek the source of immortal life.

[1] See http://en.wikipedia.org/wiki/List_of_supercentenarians; and www.grg.org/Adams/B3.HTM.

[2] For an interesting study of long-lived groups, see Dan Buettner, *The Blue Zones: Lessons for Living Longer From the People Who've Lived the Longest* (Washington, D.C.: National Geographic Society, 2008).

[3] Data from the World Health Organization, available at www.who.int/trade/glossary/story073/en/. For other figures, see International Federation of Pharmaceutical Manufacturers and Associations, "The Pharmaceutical Industry and Global Health: Facts and Figures 2012," available at www.ifpma.org/fileadmin/content/Publication/2013/IFPMA-_Facts_And_Figures_2012_LowResSinglePage.pdf.

[4] World Health Organization, "Working Together for Health," available at www.who.int/whr/2006/whr06_en.pdf?ua=1.

[5] See World Health Organization, www.who.int/mediacentre/news/releases/2014/palliative-care-20140128/en/. Map available at: www.thewpca.org/resources/global-atlas-of-palliative-care/.

[6] A. P. Carnevale et al., "Healthcare," p. 8, available at www9.georgetown.edu/grad/gpp/hpi/cew/pdfs/Healthcare.FullReport.090712.pdf.

[7] See World Economic Forum, "The Future of Pensions and Healthcare in a Rapidly Ageing World: Scenarios to 2030," available at www3.weforum.org/docs/WEF_Scenario_PensionsAndHealth2030_Report_2010.pdf.

Chapter 1

DESIGNED FOR SOMETHING BETTER

Wholeness is the Creator's gift: pursue it!

American author Annie Dillard wrote about an old woman who said: "Seem like we're just set down here," "and don't nobody know why."[1] Don't nobody know why? Even through the butchered grammar, the passion of the perennial questions—Who are we? How did we get here? How should we live? What is our purpose?—rises from her words. They are important words, too, because we can no more live a full and healthy existence without knowing its origin and purpose any more than someone who thinks an iPad's[2] just a board on which to cut radishes and onions in the kitchen could get full use out of it.

Humanity has come up with various theories and stories to explain our origins. One of the oldest teaches that some god squashed another god flat (whose body became the earth), and that each time the victorious god spit on the flattened corpse of his vanquished foe, a human appeared. On the other hand, one of the newest teaches that we don't exist at all, but are computer simulations created by a superintelligent race of aliens.

In between these two views hover others, including atheist Alex Rosenberg's claim that we exist as meaningless material entities in a meaningless material universe. "What is the purpose of the universe? There is none. What is the meaning of life? Ditto."[3] If, however, the meaninglessness of a purely materialistic universe depresses you, don't worry, because, according to Rosenberg, your depression is nothing but specific arrangements of neurons and chemicals that you can then alter with pharmaceuticals.

In contrast to the various theories and stories of how we came to be here on earth, the biblical view remains, even today (and despite endless assaults against it), the most rational, hopeful, and practical explanation for the origin and purpose of human existence. And while certainly incorporating the materialist perspective—indeed, even celebrating it—the biblical worldview isn't limited only to it, for to do so would be again like using an iPad only as a cutting board.

Intentions

In contrast to the prevailing premise of modern science that views the earth's living things as just accidents (a premise actually based on philosophy, not science), Scripture depicts the formation of life as a direct act of the Creator. In the book of Genesis everything is purposeful—nothing happens by chance. We are not simply an accidental conglomeration of randomly arranged chemicals. The formula "And God said, Let . . . and it was so" appears repeatedly throughout the Creation account in Genesis 1 and reveals direct and purposeful intentionality. Each line rejects the idea that anything is just random.

Such intentionality is especially significant when it comes to human beings. Instead of merely speaking us into existence and life, as He did all other earthly living things, God formed Adam out of the ground and then breathed into him life itself. "And the Lord God formed man of the dust of the ground, and breathed into his nostrils the breath of life; and man became a living being" (Genesis 2:7). It is an act of intimacy that, among other things, has made humanity the only being created in the "image of God" (Genesis 1:27).

Creation culminates with human existence, as if all that occurred on the five days before us were only for us. After He created humanity on the sixth day, God rested on the seventh (Genesis 2:2), because His work was done: "The heavens and the earth were finished, and all the host of them" (verse 1).

Christian author Ellen White wrote that "after the earth with its teeming animal and vegetable life had been called into existence, man, the crowning work of the Creator, and the one for whom the beautiful earth had been fitted up, was brought upon the stage of action. To him was given dominion over all that his eye could behold."[4] In contrast to the currently prevailing philosophical school of thought, one that says that we just happen to be here, we were, instead, meant to be here.

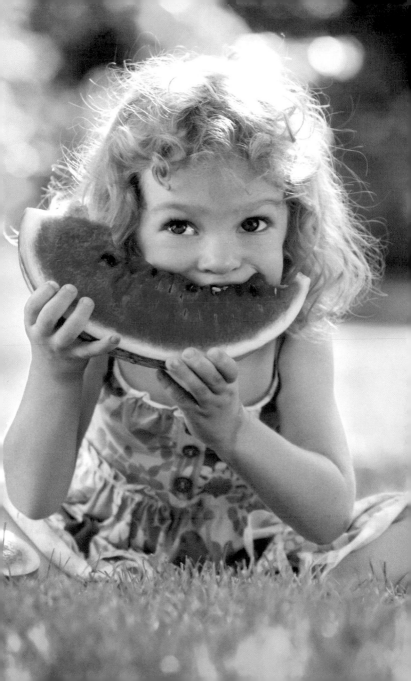

Tweaking of Dials

Though Genesis teaches that God created the earth especially for us, recent scientific discoveries have pushed that realization way beyond our planet, even to the cosmos itself. They reveal numerous finely tuned physical constants that don't allow for the slightest deviation without making our existence impossible.

For example, if the ratio between the force of electromagnetism and the force of gravity were changed by $1:10^{40}$, humans wouldn't be here. What does $1:10^{40}$ mean? Mathematician John Lennox explains: "Cover America with coins in a column reaching to the moon (236,000 miles or 380,000 kilometers away), then do the same for a billion other continents of the same size. Paint one coin red and put it somewhere in one of the billion piles. Blindfold a friend and ask her to pick it out. The odds are about 1 in 10^{40} that she will."[5]

Numerous other finely tuned factors in the cosmos, such as the distance of the earth from the sun, the speed of the earth's rotation, the energy level of carbon atoms, and the expansion rate of the universe, had to have been just right or else humanity could not have been created. Scientists have labeled these amazing ratios "anthropic coincidences"—"anthropic" from the Greek *anthropos* ("man"), and "coincidences" because, despite such mind-boggling ratios, if you rule out a Creator, what else could they be?

Nevertheless, such grossly misnamed "coincidences" help affirm what Genesis teaches: We exist in a creation that was expecting us. This point is important because foundational to our health and general happiness is a sense of meaning, of purpose. Holocaust survivor and psychiatrist Viktor Frankl argued that, at our core, we humans must find meaning to our existence or else we will live without hope, and hope is crucial to human well-being.

In short, Genesis tells us that instead of being a mere "chemical scum"[6] on the surface of the earth (Stephen Hawking), we are beings created in the image of God and we are to reflect His character and reveal His goodness and power as we ourselves marvel in that power and goodness and grow and mature in them. Created for a reason, we find meaning and purpose, including health and well-being, by seeking out and following God's intentions and desires for us.

Integrated Wholeness

Besides teaching that we were meant to be, Genesis also reveals what we are. Contrary to the ancient pagan notion that separates flesh and spirit into distinct realms (with flesh bad and spirit good), Scripture teaches what some call "an integrated wholeness," the idea that all aspects of a human being—physical, mental, and spiritual—form a single unit, and that one doesn't exist without the other. When God breathed into Adam the breath of life, the Bible doesn't say that Adam received a soul, as if it were an entity distinct from him, but that he *became* a "living soul" (*nephesh hayah*). A living soul was what he was, not what he possessed. Interestingly, the Bible uses the same phrase for the animals as well: "So God created great creatures of the sea and every living thing [*nephesh hayah*] that moves, with which the water teems and that moves about on it" (Genesis 1:21, NIV; see also verse 24). Though, obviously, different in many ways from whales and turtles, Adam was, like them, a living being, a *nephesh hayah.*

Such an understanding can protect us from two extremes. The first, a sharp dualism, emphasizes the spiritual over the physical, even to the point that it can deride the physical as evil. From Genesis onward, however, in which God deemed the completed earth as "very good" (Genesis 1:31), Scripture celebrates the physical world as a product of His creative power. Even our bodies, though fallen, are still the creations of God and need to be respected as such: "Or do you not know that your body is the temple of the Holy Spirit who is in you, whom you have from God, and you are not your own?" (1 Corinthians 6:19, NIV). The idea of our body's being bad, as opposed to a pure and eternal soul trapped in the body and eagerly awaiting release, is a pagan notion that not only makes an unwarranted division in human nature, but denies the importance of a crucial and fundamental aspect of our humanity.

The second extreme, the opposite, denies the spiritual altogether (as we saw with Alex Rosenberg) and limits all reality, including every aspect of humanity, to nothing but molecules in motion. This is, too, the philosophical presupposition, or assumption, upon which so much of modern science rests.

The biblical view, which emphasizes the reality and importance of the physical, spiritual, and mental elements of our humanity, becomes especially vital in the search for health, healing, and happiness. Our minds and bodies are inseparable aspects of our existence, and any program that seeks to bring us the best life needs to account for all aspects of our fascinatingly complicated humanity. Health includes every facet of our being. To be in good health is to be mentally alert, emotionally well adjusted, physically well, and spiritually in harmony with our Maker. Much more than the absence of disease, it involves our minds, our emotions, our bodies, and our spiritual natures.

The Miracle of Life

The complexity of our total beings prompted the psalmist to write: "I praise you because I am fearfully and wonderfully made" (Psalm 139:14, NIV). How could King David (a king, not even a physiologist) have known that he was "fearfully and wonderfully" made? The man wrote almost 3,000 years ago, long before microscopes and X-ray machines, much less CAT scans and MRIs. David didn't have a clue what a cell was, much less about any of its myriad and fantastically complicated parts. What did he know about cell reproduction or protein synthesis? He wouldn't have even recognized what a protein was.

David never heard of DNA, and his mind certainly couldn't understand (neither can ours, actually) how a single human body has 20 trillion meters of DNA , and that our complete set of genes (the genome) is more than 3.5 billion letters long. What did he know about how white blood cells fight invaders, or about the many steps in the enzyme cascade that leads to blood clotting?

Nevertheless, he knew enough to realize what a miracle it was that we exist, and enough to praise the God who brought about that existence.

Wholeness in a Broken World

However wonderfully made, we are still fallen beings in a fallen world (see Genesis 3), and as such we are susceptible to sickness, pain, and death. In the end, only the redemption found in Jesus, climaxing at the Second Coming, will bring full restoration and healing to us. Until then, "our first duty toward God and our fellow beings is that of self-development. Every faculty with which the Creator has endowed us should be cultivated to the highest degree of perfection, that we may be able to do the greatest amount of good of which we are capable. Hence that time is spent to good account which is used in the establishment and preservation of physical and mental health."[7]

Without question, the old woman who spoke to Annie Dillard had it right: we have been "set down here." But her "and don't nobody know why" phrase missed the mark completely. We do know why. We were "set down here" because, as the Bible says, God has "made us, and not we ourselves" (Psalm 100:3). Yes, God made us, molding Adam out of "the dust of the ground" and then breathing life and consciousness into that molded dust, and he became "a living soul." God brought us into being for a purpose: to enjoy life in all of its fullness and richness, and to know the love of God in all of its beauty. In every heart there exists an aching void that only He can fill. When He occupies that emptiness within, He becomes the real purpose for living, and our joy is complete.

Our existence is a miracle, and our life a precious gift (just ask someone who is losing it). And, as with all precious gifts, we must cherish it and care for it, which includes doing our best to develop and maintain the physical, mental, and spiritual components of a human being fashioned in the image of God. We are stewards of the gift of life. There is no more precious gift and no more important task than living a life of abundant health so that we can honor our Creator, serve others, and experience life to the full.

[1] Annie Dillard, *The Annie Dillard Reader* (New York: HarperCollins, 1994), p. 281.

[2] An iPad is a type of tablet computer that is smaller than a laptop computer and utilized by touching icons on its screen rather than using a keyboard. A company called Apple developed it.

[3] Alex Rosenberg, *The Atheist's Guide to Reality: Enjoying Life Without Illusions* (New York: W. W. Norton, 2011), p. 2.

[4] Ellen G. White, *Patriarchs and Prophets* (Mountain View, Calif.: Pacific Press Pub. Assn., 1890), p. 44.

[5] John Lennox, *God's Undertaker: Has Science Buried God?* (Kindle edition), p. 71.

[6] Stephen Hawking, quoted in David Deutsch, *The Fabric of Reality: The Science of Parallel Universes—and Its Implications* (New York: Penguin, 1997), pp. 177, 178.

[7] Ellen G. White, *Counsels on Health* (Mountain View, Calif.: Pacific Press Pub. Assn., 1923), p. 107.

Chapter 2

DIET FOR A LIFETIME

Wholesome food strengthens healthy bodies: enjoy it.

Let's suppose you just purchased the car of your dreams: a Porsche Panamera, a Mercedes-Benz S-Class, or an Audi A8. Would you even think of using the lowest grade of fuel possible, neglecting to change the oil, or totally ignoring all of the manufacturer's suggested maintenance checks? Certainly not! If you had just paid more than $90,000 for a luxury car, you would be extremely conscientious about keeping it in optimum condition.

The human body is far more beautiful, complex, and finely tuned than any automobile in the world. Our bodies are a marvel of infinite engineering intelligence. Think of the wonders of a single cell, the complexity of the brain, the intricacies of the heart, or the divine miracle of birth. We stand amazed at the carefully crafted design of the human body. A loving Creator went to infinite lengths to create us, and, like a luxury car, our bodies also the best possible fuel to power our lives, and that fuel comes from the food we eat. Without premium fuel in a luxury car the mileage goes down, power is lost, and the engine does not run as smoothly. And without the right nutrition, our bodies just do not function properly either.

A balanced diet chosen from the best foods will provide the essential nutrients needed for growth, maintenance, and energy. When we pick low-quality foods or don't eat enough of even the best foods, the body machinery suffers. And if we overeat highly refined foods, we can easily become overweight and lack vital nutrients. The One who made us cares about our health, and so should we. The apostle John certainly echoed the desire of our Lord's heart when he prayed, "Beloved, I pray that you may prosper in all things and be in health, just as your soul prospers" (3 John 2, NKJV).

Caring for our bodies is not something we do in addition to being a Christian. It is at the heart of God's plan for our lives. Do not misunderstand. We cannot eat our way into heaven. We are saved by grace and grace alone (Ephesians 2:8). However, we may fail to achieve God's purpose for our lives because our poor eating habits bring premature and preventable disease and death. Make no mistake about it: What we eat is important.

Understanding Good Nutrition

We fuel our bodies from the foods we choose to eat. They provide the nutrients essential for a healthy and productive life. Digestion is the intricate process of breaking down food into its individual building blocks so that the body can assimilate and use them to sustain life. This process begins in the mouth, moves to the stomach, then to the small intestines, and finally to the large bowel.

We can divide the nutrients our bodies need into these important categories:

- **Carbohydrates:** In a "premium fuel" diet, the largest portion of carbohydrates should come from rich unrefined sources, such as whole grains, legumes, fruits, and vegetables.
- **Proteins:** Every cell in the body contains proteins. Tissue repair and growth require them. While almost all foods have some protein, animal products such as milk and eggs are also good sources, but not the only ones. Legumes (beans) contain excellent protein.
- **Fats:** These are concentrated sources of energy. We often get too much fat in our diet because we like the flavor it imparts to foods. Many people would rather eat French fries than boiled potatoes. Nuts in moderate amounts provide excellent quality fats, however. The body needs such fats to absorb fat-soluble vitamins.
- **Vitamins:** These are essential organic components of the diet, and are required in small amounts for normal growth and activity. Most occur naturally in various foods. Some are fat-soluble and others water-soluble, and when we do not have a sufficient supply, a deficiency results.
- **Minerals:** These inorganic elements are vital to human health and are easily obtained from both animal and plant foods. Too little of them can lead to a deficiency.

- **Antioxidants and phytochemicals:** Scientists now recognize hundreds of these substances, which protect the body from disease and some of the effects of aging. We find them primarily in whole grains, fruits, vegetables, and nuts.

You need all these categories of food in order to enjoy good health. The secret is in their combination.

Abundant Nutrition From a Simple Food Plan

What is the best diet for optimum health? Think of the diet that God gave to our first parents in the Garden of Eden. In the Bible's first book, Genesis, God Himself offers us a menu for good health. "And God said, 'See, I have given you every herb that yields seed which is on the face of all the earth, and every tree whose fruit yields seed; to you it shall be for food' " (Genesis 1:29, NKJV). The Creator's original diet was a plant-based one. When Adam and Eve left the garden, our Lord added the "herb of the field" (Genesis 3:18, NKJV), or the root vegetables, to their daily fare. By basing our diet on foods wisely chosen in appropriate amounts from the Master's menu, we can easily meet our optimal nutrient needs:

- **Cereals and grains:** These should form the foundation of our diet; they include whole-grain breads, pastas, rice, and corn. When chosen from unrefined (not white) sources, each is rich in dietary fiber, complex carbohydrates, and an array of vitamins and minerals.
- **Fruits and vegetables:** These foods come in a wide variety of colors, flavors, and textures, and are the richest sources of protective phytochemicals, antioxidants, vitamins, and minerals. Many people seem to prefer fruits to vegetables, but we need a balance of both. Foods in this group that are the deepest in color often have the largest amounts of phytochemicals and antioxidants.
- **Legumes, nuts, and seeds:** Legumes, such as beans, peas, and lentils, are an excellent source of good protein, along with minerals, vitamins, and other protective elements. Nuts and seeds provide essential fats, but because they're a concentrated source of calories, we should limit them to no more than one to two servings per day. Nonvegetarians would include fish, fowl, and meat in this group, but these, if consumed at all, should

be eaten in moderate amounts only. Some choose to include dairy and eggs in their diets. It is important to recognize that all animal products are high in cholesterol, which may contribute to coronary artery disease. Although animal sources of food provide many important nutrients, including calcium and vitamin B_{12}, they do pose some health risks. Vitamin B_{12} appears only in animal products and prevents pernicious anemia and neurological disorders, as well as promoting normal cellular division. It's vital that those who choose not to consume any animal products to include sufficient foods fortified with vitamin B_{12} or to get it in supplement form on a regular basis.

- **Fats, oils, sweets, and salt:** The body needs such foods only in small amounts.

While the essential fats and sodium are vital for optimum health, excessive amounts can cause serious health problems. Iodine is a necessary trace mineral easily obtained if one uses iodized salt, but it can also be gotten from sea salt, seaweed, or a supplement. We do not require refined sugar for good health, but small amounts add palatability and flavor to food. Nutritional scientists today recognize that plant foods should form the foundation of healthful eating to sustain good health and reduce the risk of disease. One of the most important keys to eating a balanced plant-based diet is selecting a variety of foods whose color, texture, and flavor add interest to the diet. Such foods are best when consumed as they come from nature: not refined or broken down. Whole foods should be the goal.

Today medical science recognizes the advantages of a vegetarian diet. A plant-based vegetarian diet is:

- low in fat, particularly saturated fat
- low in refined sugar
- lacking cholesterol (with a total vegetarian diet)
- high in dietary fiber
- high in protective phytochemicals, antioxidants, etc.
- rich in sources of vitamins and minerals

Having stressed the advantages of adopting certain categories of food, especially a vegetarian diet, we now turn our attention to knowing what to take into account when selecting foods.

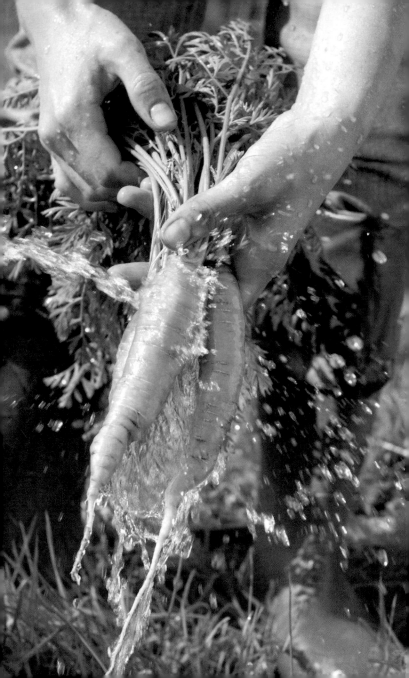

Principles for Healthful Food Choices

A healthful diet requires good food choices. Keep in mind the following simple principles:

- **Variety:** The most important principle of eating well is selecting a variety of foods. This ensures a wide range of nutrients to support a healthy body, and the various textures, tastes, and colors enhance the pleasure of eating.

- **Quality:** Choose the majority of your food from whole foods, not refined ones. Such foods are nutrient-dense rather than calorie-dense.

- **Moderation:** Some important components of a healthful diet we should eat only in small amounts. Our bodies require adequate amounts of the essential fats as well as small amounts of salt to maintain our electrolytes. But obesity is a growing problem worldwide. It's even possible to eat too much good food! We must balance the amount of energy we consume with the energy we expend in physical activity if we are to remain at a healthful weight.

- **Avoidance:** Highly refined foods that often have large amounts of their nutritional elements removed should be avoided, as should foods and beverages that have no nutritional value (for example, alcohol, coffee, and sodas).

Some people eat as though they don't believe it makes any difference what they consume. But it does. Dr. Gary Fraser, an eminent cardiologist and research scientist, explains how dietary choices and lifestyle affect our longevity and quality of life: "Early in my career as a scientist and physician the great advantages of prevention rather than waiting to treat established disease became clear. Despite the great advances of modern medicine, the expense, sometimes discomfort, and lack of assurance of cure make medical treatment an inferior approach to the control of disease. . . . My colleagues and I have had the opportunity to collect data that in a rigorous scientific fashion allow us to investigate the value of a vegetarian diet. After many years of research by us (and other groups), the evidence is now clear. A plant-based diet provides a host of advantages over a diet containing much meat, as is commonly consumed among our neighbors in the United States and in many other parts of the world.

"We now know," he continues, "and have published evidence in medical journals, that American vegetarian Adventists, as compared to nonvegetarian Adventists, have less hypertension, lower LDL [bad] cholesterol, lower levels of fasting sugar and insulin, lower levels of C-reactive protein [a chemical that is associated with inflammation], less diabetes, and much less of a problem with overweight and obesity. In addition, there is clear evidence of moderately lower mortality among Adventist vegetarians when compared to nonvegetarians. This is particularly from cardiovascular disease and diabetes/kidney disease. The frequency of certain cancers also appears to be less among vegetarians."

According to Dr. Fraser, studies of 34,000 Californian Adventists back in the 1980s and 1990s demonstrated that as a group Adventist men lived more than seven years and women more than four years longer than their non-Adventist neighbors, making them one of the longest-lived populations ever reported. The *National Geographic* has cited Loma Linda, California (actually representing Californian Adventists), as the American "blue zone," a term used to refer to an area of unusual longevity. "Just as important," says Dr. Fraser, "we also have demonstrated across the country that at each decade of life Adventists enjoy better physical and mental quality of life than their non-Adventist peers. Thus, it appears that the extra years of life are generally good-quality years."

Dr. Fraser's observation speaks to each one of our desires. Each of us desires "good-quality years." We want to add not only years to our life, but life to our years. What would a few more years be if they were absolutely miserable? That is why Jesus instructed us that "man shall not live by bread alone, but by every word that proceedeth out of the mouth of God" (Matthew 4:4). God's words give us hope and courage to face life's most difficult challenges. They offer us a new peace and purpose for living.

The Old Testament prophet Jeremiah cries out, "Your words were found, and I ate them, and Your word was to me the joy and rejoicing of my heart; for I am called by Your name, O Lord God of hosts" (Jeremiah 15:16, NKJV). Just as good nutritious food nourishes our bodies, God's Word nourishes our souls.

Deep within each one of us there lurks a soul hunger to know the truth about life's meaning and purpose. As we have seen already, the Bible reveals where we came from, why we are here, and where we are going. It tells us that we were created by a loving God who cares for us more than we can imagine. He is a God who will never leave us or forsake us but wants us in heaven even more than we desire to be there. The Bible portrays a God of incredible hope who is preparing an eternal banquet for us one day soon in eternity. Until then, He invites us to care for our bodies here in anticipation of living with Him in the earth made new. Therefore, dedicate your body to God and choose to honor Him in the things that you eat and drink. You can look forward to one day sitting around a throne and eating with God at the royal banquet in His kingdom.

Chapter 3

ARE YOU AT RISK?

Obesity, which causes several diseases,
need not be devastating: understand it.

Joe was tired and short of breath. Even the simplest physical tasks, such as walking around the house or to the car, left him breathing hard. He sat in the doctor's office, discouraged and distressed. He had not lost any weight since his previous visit two months before. To complicate matters, he was still smoking, and his blood sugar tests were way above normal. But he still could not resist the sugary doughnuts that he would eat each morning, washed down with sugary-sweet coffee or cola drinks. As a result of his type 2 diabetes, smoking, obesity, and very sedentary lifestyle, Joe had experienced his first heart attack two years before, at age 35. It was a massive one, leaving him with a big scar on his heart muscle and heart failure.

A little embarrassed, Joe nervously expressed his concerns to his physician. "Well, Doc, I knew you would not be happy with my lack of progress in getting my weight down, and because I still smoke cigarettes a little—mind you, I don't inhale! Sorry, Doc; I don't want to disappoint you."

The doctor kindly encouraged him to keep trying, pointing out that with the damage the heart attack had caused to the pumping ability of the heart, the uncontrolled diabetes, the ongoing cigarette use, and his overweight, if he did not make drastic changes he would die at a young age.

Joe's response was quite remarkable: "How about a heart transplant, Doc? I've heard about them. Can I get a new heart?"

"I wish it were as easy and simple as that," his physician said. "Donor hearts are in short supply, and then there is all the medication for years afterward. It is a last resort that may help, but one limited to the very few. You must make lifestyle changes—and right away." Finally Joe understood the seriousness of his condition and started reshaping how he lived.

Millions of men and women just like Joe struggle all around the world with noncommunicable diseases: heart conditions, cancers, respiratory diseases, and diabetes. They share four main risk factors: tobacco use, physical inactivity, alcohol, and unhealthy diets. You may be at risk and not fully realize it.

The Obesity Pandemic

The problem of overweight and obesity has become so wide-spread that health professionals have begun calling it a pandemic. When any disease reaches high levels in a community or geographic area, medical science refers to it as an *epidemic*, but when it occurs in many parts of the world at the same time, it's termed *pandemic*.

According to the World Health Organization, at least 2.8 million people die worldwide each year as a direct result of being overweight or obese. It strikes rich and poor countries alike. Obesity is no longer a characteristic of high-income societies.

You can calculate the amount of overweight or obesity, usually defined as "abnormal or excessive fat accumulation that may impair health," by finding your body mass index (BMI). To do the math, divide your weight in pounds by the square of your height in inches then multiply that answer by 703. If your BMI is equal to or more than 25, you are overweight, and if it is equal to or more than 30, you have obesity. In either case, it is good to start a program of lifestyle changes.

The formula in metric units is: BMI = (weight in kilograms) / (height in meters x height in meters). For example, if you weigh 60 kilograms and are 1.70 meters high, the BMI will be:

BMI = 60 / (1.7 x 1.7) = 20.8 (you are in the normal category).

If you do not want to bother to make the calculations, just go to the Internet for a BMI calculator. You will find many, both in English and metric units.[1]

What does your BMI say? Are you at risk? Are you overweight? Is your blood pressure normal? Do you eat large servings of fatty, high-calorie, refined, and processed foods? Does your diet come mainly from fast-food outlets? If so, you're headed for trouble, or

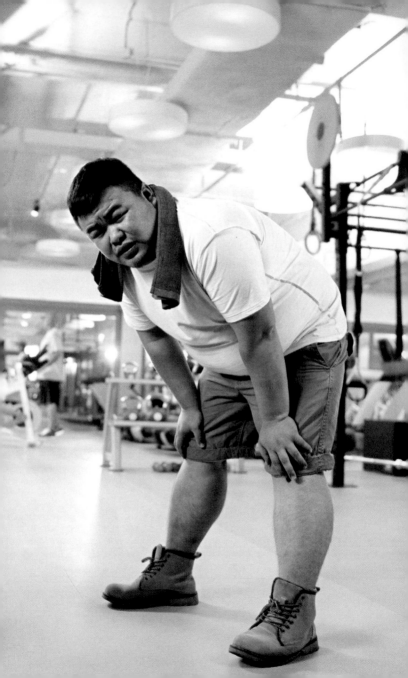

BMI classification	
Underweight	<18.5
Normal range	18.5—24.9
Overweight	≥25.0
Preobese	25.0—29.9
Obese	≥30.0
Obese class I	30.0—39.9
Obese class II	35.0—39.9
Obese class III	≥40.0

you may already have problems with your health and not be aware of it.

The media advertises many "miraculous" plans for losing weight, but the best and safest is a radical change in lifestyle as proposed in this book.

Obesity + Diabetes = "Diabesity"

Several health problems result from obesity, including increased risk of heart disease, high blood pressure, and certain cancers. Yet one of the more common is diabetes, which we will focus on here. More than one third of a billion people in the world have diabetes—about one of every 20 people on earth! The countries with the largest likely diabetes increase by 2030 include China, India, and the United States. They all lead many others, both rich and poor.[2] Obesity, defined as a person weighing 20 percent or more above the normal weight for their height, is the number one risk factor for developing type 2 diabetes. As many as 80 percent of people with type 2 diabetes are obese. The two conditions of diabetes and obesity are so closely linked that many health experts refer to them as one disease, which they have dubbed *diabesity*.

The rate of diabetes has risen dramatically in the general population in recent years, as has the incidence of obesity, the number one risk factor for diabetes. An estimated 3.4 million people worldwide die from the complications of diabetes each year. The World Health Organization projects that diabetes will be the seventh-leading cause of death by the year 2030.[3] If diabetes is such a mortal enemy, then it is important to know how to overcome it.

What Is Diabetes?

Running through our bodies is an intricate system of blood vessels that we can think of as pipes ranging in size from about one inch (2.5 centimeters) to as small as .0002 inches, just enough room for one red blood cell to squeeze through at a time. The blood carries all the nutrients needed by every cell in your body to perform their correct functions. The energy source for cells is a simple form of sugar called *glucose.* Too much glucose (sugar) can damage the cells. The body, therefore, has an amazing way of regulating the amount of sugar in the blood. It does so by *insulin*, a substance produced by cells in the pancreas.

Diabetes is a chronic disease in which the amount of sugar carried in the blood does not get regulated as it should be. Either the body does not produce insulin normally (type 1 diabetes, also known as T1DM), or it develops resistance to insulin, which means the sugar is not effectively controlled (type 2 diabetes, or T2DM).

A third type of diabetes can develop in pregnant women who have not had diabetes before. It most often occurs after three months of pregnancy. Obesity in pregnancy is a leading risk factor for child-hood obesity. It also increases the potential for high blood pressure during pregnancy, as well as other severe complications of pregnancy. Babies born to obese mothers are more likely to have birth defects and heart problems.[4]

Diabesity during pregnancy can lead to significant complications for both mother and child. High maternal blood glucose damages the delicate functioning of the baby's cells, which leads to cell death and increased abnormalities in the child.

People who have diabetes often complain of passing markedly in-creased amounts of urine. The high levels of sugar in the blood spill over into the urine. The increased fluid (and sugar) loss through urine stimulates the thirst mechanism, causing them to drink a lot of water to compensate. Body weight may decrease, and long-term damage to nerves and blood vessels (the latter injury can lead to heart attack, stroke, and kidney failure) may result. The destruction of neglected blood vessels can cause gangrene of the limbs.

Prevention, Reversal, or Control of Diabetes

Careful blood sugar control helps prevent the negative effects of diabesity and improves pregnancy outcomes, but it can be difficult to achieve. A diet low in refined carbohydrates and saturated fat, com-bined with moderate exercise, can improve the health of the mother and baby, because such lifestyle changes help control weight during pregnancy. For women who are morbidly (very) obese and contemplating pregnancy, surgical interventions can be helpful alternatives to diet and exercise to regulate weight and prevent onset of, or reverse, diabetes. Through rigorous monitoring and strict adherence to health plans, it *is* possible to avert diabesity and its complications.

Diabetics must carefully control their blood sugar levels and sometimes may require insulin (injections)—most commonly in type 1 diabetes. Some patients with type 2 diabetes require sugar-lowering tablets, but the mainstay of treatment is changing to a plant-based diet rich in fresh fruit, fresh vegetables, and nuts, and low in refined carbohydrates and saturated fats. Lifestyle changes such as exercise and weight loss can prevent or delay the onset of type 2 diabetes.

The American Diabetes Association discussed the value of a plant-based diet and made this observation: "A vegetarian diet is a healthy option, even if you have diabetes. Research supports that following this type of diet can help prevent and manage diabetes. . . . Vegan diets [a total plant-based diet] are naturally higher in fiber, much lower in saturated fat, and cholesterol-free when compared to a traditional American diet. . . . The high fiber in this diet may help you feel full for a longer time after eating and may help you eat less over time. . . . This diet also tends to cost less. Meat, poultry, and fish are usually the most expensive foods we eat."[5]

Such lifestyle measures bring huge benefits and are not too expensive. While they demand commitment and time, they do help to keep the blood glucose close to normal and prevent damage to the eyes, kidneys, and blood vessels—especially of the lower limbs. British physician and researcher Denis Burkitt was right when he commented, "If people are constantly falling off a cliff, you could place ambulances under the cliff or build a fence on the top of the cliff. We are placing all too many ambulances under the cliff."

Many people are essentially saying, "Doc, let me live like I want, eat what I want, smoke and drink what I want, then give me a magic pill to keep me well." But there is a much better way than disregarding the laws of health and hoping beyond hope to stay well. Instead, we can build "fences" to protect ourselves and our children against premature disease and death by eating a healthy natural diet, exercising regularly, getting adequate rest, drinking plenty of water, developing positive relationships, and having faith in a God who really cares for us. We have an enormous challenge and also a great opportunity. Prevention is preferable to an ambulance. It is not only better than the cure—it *is* the cure. As adults, we have the privilege of modeling healthful behaviors for our children that will protect them from the raging pandemic.

At the same time, our own health will benefit. We need to be physically active and encourage our children to exercise too. We must be responsible architects of their choices, providing the most healthful food options as priorities in our budgets. That applies especially to pregnant mothers, who shape both their children's choices and their own future health, or possible lack thereof.

The Bible has great advice and encouragement for guiding our children's as well as our own decisions in health and general behaviors: "Start children off on the way they should go, and even when they are old they will not turn from it" (Proverbs 22:6, NIV). We see the importance of repetition in instruction and example well described in the following advice regarding God's law and directions: "These commandments that I give you today are to be on your hearts. Impress them on your children. Talk about them when you sit at home and when you walk along the road, when you lie down and when you get up" (Deuteronomy 6:6, 7, NIV). As parents we need to invest time, love, example, and perseverance from conception of the baby until the child becomes independent of parental care.

Scripture reminds that we are "fearfully and wonderfully made" (Psalm 139:14). Our response of praise and gratitude, therefore, should be to honor our Creator in all things: "Whether you eat or drink or whatever you do, do it all for the glory of God" (1 Corinthians 10:31, NIV). He is faithful in helping to guide our decisions and choices from portion sizes and the foods best suited to our needs, to exercise and adequate rest. One of the greatest motivations to keep our bodies in good health is to honor the God who created us. There is something much more than merely being healthy for health's sake, as important as that is, or a personal desire to live longer on earth. Even if we meticulously follow the laws of health, all of us will die sometime unless our Lord returns first. Our bodies are not a fun house. They are the temples of the Holy Spirit, and that makes all the difference.

A number of years ago Dr. Albert Reece, dean of the School of Medicine at the University of Maryland, was helping a woman who had smoked for decades to quit. He tried everything, but she just could not seem to stop. She might be off cigarettes for a few days, but then would start smoking again. One day Dr. Reece, who is a Christian, shared the fact that her body was the temple of the Holy Spirit and that Jesus through the Holy Spirit longed to dwell in her body. He explained that the choices she made in caring for her body would determine in part her fitness for eternity. A week or so later, when he visited her to offer encouragement, she said, "I quit. I have not smoked since our last visit. When I wanted to take a puff, I pictured the Holy Spirit choking. I no longer desire to defile my body temple with tobacco. I want to present my body to Jesus in the best possible condition when He returns."

Would you like to offer your body as a living sacrifice to Jesus as His temple to dwell in by His Holy Spirit? Why don't you invite Him right now to strengthen your resolve and commitment to healthful living? He will immediately come to your aid. If you need a change of heart by the Great Physician, God can do it, as the Bible says in Ezekiel 36:26: "I will give you a new heart and put a new spirit in you. . . . I will move you to follow my decrees and be careful to keep my laws" (NIV). We all need help to make changes in our behavior. Look for help outside of yourself—seek God's help. You cannot do it without Him, but He will not do it without your choice and co-operation. Ask a close friend or family member to partner with you and encourage accountability and pray together. You'll be glad you did as you experience positive results and live life to the full!

[1] For example, www.nhlbi.nih.gov/guidelines/obesity/BMI/bmicalc.htm.

[2] S. Wild, G. Roglic, A. Green, R. Sicree, H. King, "Global Prevalence of Diabetes: Estimates for the Year 2000 and Projections for 2030," *Diabetes Care* 27 (2004): 1047-1053.

[3] World Health Organization, "Fact Sheet No. 312," available online at www.who.int/mediacentre/factsheets/fs312/en/.

[4] K. J. Stothard et al., "Maternal Overweight and Obesity and the Risk of Congenital Anomalies: A Systematic Review and Meta-analysis," *JAMA* 301 (2009): 636-650.

[5] Available online at www.diabetes.org/food-and-fitness/food/planning-meals-meal-planning-for-vegetarians/.

Chapter 4

FIT FOR LIFE

Exercise is a choice: practice it.

Excitement filled the air. The enthusiastic crowd cheered wildly as Roger Bannister sprinted around the Iffley Track Road in Oxford, England. Bannister had meticulously prepared for the race. Totally focused on his goal of breaking the four-minute mile, he followed an extremely disciplined training regime. The preparation was intense and even included rigorous mountain climbing. While Bannister was obviously seeking to break this elusive record, others around the world also had their eyes on the same goal.

May 6, 1954, dawned, and Roger Bannister knew that it was the day he had been working toward emotionally, spiritually, intellectually, and physically. On May 5 he had slipped on a polished floor in the hospital and limped the rest of the day. Doubts, questions, determination, and excited anticipation filled his mind in the run up to the race. Then, paced by his two colleagues Chris Brasher and Chris Chataway, Bannister ran the mile in 3 minutes and 59.4 seconds! He pressed toward the mark and won the prize—the coveted record of the first man to run the under-four-minute mile! It demanded discipline for Roger Bannister to achieve his goal.

Most things that are worthwhile take effort, and that is especially true of our health. Good health is not something that comes by some stroke of luck. It is not a matter of chance. Although each one of us has different genetic makeups and predispositions to disease, following the principles of health that our Creator has written on every nerve and tissue of our bodies contributes to our overall well-being. When you have worked all day and are just about worn out, it takes real discipline to exercise. Or when you are tired and would much rather munch on peanuts while watching your favorite comedy on television, it takes a determined choice to get off the couch and exercise. Now, don't misunderstand. We are not encouraging you to be "Roger Bannister the second." Your goal is not to try to run the four-minute mile tomorrow. It is to evaluate where you are, consult with your health-care provider, and begin regular, systematic exercise appropriate for your age and abilities. For some younger people it may be more vigorous than for those of us who are a little older.

What will it take to motivate you to begin and maintain a regular exercise program? If you aren't regularly exercising now, what will it require to get you going?

Exercise Essentials

Exercise is one way to start your body moving in the direction of good health. The father of medicine, Hippocrates, once said, "If we could give every individual the right amount of nourishment and exercise, not too little and not too much, we would have found the safest way to health." That is also our challenge in the twenty-first century. Most of us stare at one screen after another—smartphones, iPads, e-readers, and computers—up to eight hours a day. Then, if you add TV watching, we end up spending more time in front of screens than we do sleeping! With continued mechanization, even manual occupations require less physical activity. Vibrant health requires activity, movement, and exercise. Good health isn't only about not being ill—it's about being happy and feeling whole from a physical, mental, social, and spiritual point of view. Exercise and activity help to make those outcomes a reality.

Above all, exercise is a part of the total health package. Ellen White, an inspired health educator, outlined a balanced, multifaceted approach to healthful living that has stood the test of time and science: "Pure air, sunlight, abstemiousness, rest, exercise, proper diet, the use of water, trust in divine power—these are the true remedies. Every person should have a knowledge of nature's remedial agencies and how to apply them."[1]

The goal of exercise is to maintain or enhance our overall physical fitness and general health. People exercise to strengthen muscles, optimize the cardiovascular system, control body weight, develop

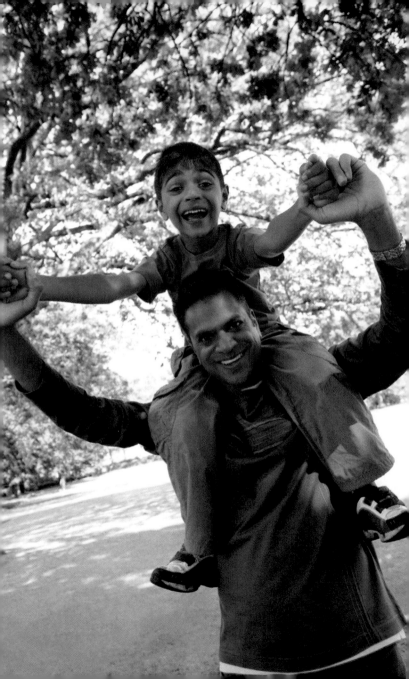

athletic skills, improve physical appearance, facilitate general well-ness and mental alertness, and also to socialize and have fun. It is the single most important thing we can do to enhance our longevity.

Ellen White offers another helpful perspective. "The body is the only medium through which the mind and the soul are developed for the up building of character."[2] In the same way that a good foundation is the basis of a building structure, a well-functioning body facilitates the development of one's mental capabilities and, ultimately, one's character.

Benefits of Exercise

Unless you overexercise or exercise in the wrong manner, physical activity is always beneficial. It's never too late to start, and some exercise is better than none at all.

Exercise facilitates sustainable weight loss and improves posture and appearance. It also reduces the risk and the progression of heart disease, diabetes, cancer, and Alzheimer's, as well as premature death. Have you ever felt stiff and wished you had more flexibility? Exercise increases body flexibility, strengthens bones and joints, protects against fractures, and builds healthy muscles. The benefits that follow exercise include lowered blood pressure, lowered heart rate, and a decreased risk for both obesity and diabetes. If you feel too tired to exercise, remember that exercise increases energy, vitality, speed, and performance. Fitness facilitates recovery from injury and illness.

Now that we have considered the physical benefits of exercise, what about its mental benefits? If ever there existed a magic formula for health, it is exercise. A good walk in the park or jog around the block improves learning, retention, and overall mental function. It is a great stress reliever and enhances overall psychological health. The rates of depression decrease, and self-esteem increases in those who exercise. Have you ever noticed that when you have exercised that day you sleep better?

Exercise also provides some surprising social benefits. It facilitates emotional intelligence and conflict resolution, strengthens intimacy and sexual life, and promotes feelings of happiness. Since exercise increases the flow of oxygen carrying blood cells to the brain, it also enhances our ability to meditate, pray, and study the Bible. Systematic exercise increases our capacity to appreciate spiritual things. With the renewed energy that comes from exercise we will also have a greater desire to serve others.

A Plan and Pointers

One of the world's leading professional organizations in exercise physiology, the American College of Sports Medicine, has designed a template for a healthy amount of exercise. We each need at least 150 minutes of moderate exercise per week. For most, this is a very reachable goal. All that we need is a sidewalk, a trail in the woods, a treadmill—and a small time commitment that adds up to fewer than three hours a week, or about 30 minutes a day, for exercise. Surprisingly enough, you do not need to be a world-class sprinter or weight lifter to get enough exercise. A brisk walk for a minimum of 30 minutes five times a week will do. Recent research indicates that we do not need to take the exercise all at one time. Three 10-minute sessions will give the same benefits that 30 minutes will confer.

Of course, it's not enough just to read and talk about exercise—you must do it! Someone has said, "All the talking about walking will not take the place of a good walk." Review your past habits, assess what they are now, and decide what you want them to be. Don't worry about whether you'll be successful or not. Simply determine to do your best from this point forward. Then start.

1. Plan: While there are many exercise programs available, here are four principles to keep in mind: the frequency and intensity of your exercise program, along with the time and type of your exercise regime. But always consult with your physician before starting it. Let's look briefly at each of the four components of a good exercise program.

- **Frequency** has to do with how often you exercise. For cardio exercise, most exercise specialists suggest moderate exercise five days a week or intense cardio three days a week to improve your health. For weight loss, you may need to do up to six or more days a week. And for strength training, the recommended frequency is two or three nonconsecutive days a week with at least a one- or two-day break between sessions.

- **Intensity** involves how hard you exercise. The general rule for cardio exercise is to work in your target heart-rate zone and focus on a variety of intensities to stimulate different energy systems. For strength training, the exercises you do, the amount of weight you lift, and your sets and repetitions determine the intensity of your workouts.

- **Time** concerns how long you should exercise. Exercise guidelines suggest that your goal should be 30-60 minutes per session. That does not mean you will start by exercising for an hour. It may take you some time to work your way up to that level of cardio exercise. Begin slowly. If you have not been exercising for a while, you cannot make up for 10 years of lack of it in one day. Its intensity and your fitness level will determine the duration of your exercise. The harder you work, the shorter your workouts will be.

- For cardio exercise you can do any **type** of activity that increases your heart rate, such as running, walking, cycling, swimming, sports, etc. Strength training includes basically any exercise with which you're using some form of resistance (bands, dumbbells, machines, etc.) to work your muscles.

Remember these four principles:

a. Frequency: exercise regularly.

b. Intensity: exercise strenuously.

c. Time: exercise at least 30 minutes a day.

d. Type: incorporate both aerobic exercise and strength-building exercise into your exercise program.

As you follow this basic exercise outline, it will help you to adjust your workouts to avoid boredom, overuse injuries, and weight-loss plateaus.

The simplest measure of adequate aerobic exercise is to obtain a pedometer (step counter) and walk the recommended 10,000 steps per day every day! This will ensure basic personal fitness.

2. Pointers: In order for your program to work regardless of whether you're a beginner or a "pro," here are some helpful pointers.

- Move. Nothing will happen unless you take action. Just do it!
- Use the three-step change model. First, know where you are now; second, decide where you want to be; third, develop a plan to get there.
- Learn more about exercises. Begin to research subjects related to your particular interests. Emphasize the positive aspects of practicing a healthful lifestyle—think it, believe it, talk it. Start and restart with the belief that you will be successful.
- Evaluate your performance. Some people find it helpful to keep a log of when they start exercising, then make notes of their progress (you will find many good exercise logs available on the Internet to assist you).
- Get moving. Start today and don't stop. Continuity is essential. Remember that the three major exercise stoppers are: (a) procrastination, (b) lack of persistence, and (c) self-defeating attitudes. You may not achieve all of your goals, but do not become discouraged. Never give up on your exercise.

Remember that all the good you do for your body will only complement and support your spiritual and mental objectives. Exercise, and relish the positive feelings that it brings. Evaluate your progress and remain motivated.

Extra Strength

Good religion is complemented by good health habits, which, of necessity, should include exercise. The body and soul are wedded to each other, and it's proper to pray that they both may prosper to the glory of God. "Beloved, I pray that you may prosper in all things and be in health, just as your soul prospers" (3 John 1:2, NKJV). Whenever we face problems, obstacles, or challenges in doing God's will, including exercising, we have the privilege of asking Him for help to strengthen our resolve. As we choose to live in harmony with the principles of positive, healthful living, He will strengthen us to do the right thing. We're not in this battle alone. You can do all things through Christ, who strengthens you (see Philippians 4:13).

Your body is the temple of God, through which He communicates. Exercise helps to keep that temple in good shape so that you can perceive what God wants you to do, and then be able to do it. Many people overeat, have bad habits, and don't exercise. Then they pray that God may heal their bodies. Isn't it rather presumptuous of us to think that we can knowingly violate the laws of health and expect God to give us good health? Although exercise will not guarantee good health, not exercising may very well guarantee we will not have it.

Each day, plan to spend some time in exercise. Use this time to breathe a prayer and fellowship with your Maker. It will invigorate your mind, body, and spirit. With exercising and good health there's no room for excuses and procrastination. We have to make it happen to maintain health and wellness. No one can do it for you but you. Now it's up to you!

[1] E. G. White, *Counsels on Health*, p. 90.
[2] Ellen G. White, *My Life Today* (Washington, D.C.: Review and Herald Pub. Assn., 1952), p. 78.

Chapter 5

HEALTHY RELATIONSHIPS

Love matters: invest in it.

Esther sat in the consulting room, slumped in her chair. Although she was only 24 years old, sadness darkened her eyes. Something or someone had robbed her joy. Reluctantly she acknowledged that she had many health problems, but had never seen a doctor. She described how both of her parents had beaten her for wetting her bed since the age of 3. As she grew older, the incontinent episodes continued, and so did the beatings. The fear of being hurt for something beyond her control intensified. When Esther became an adolescent, she still had problems controlling her bladder, and she also experienced unpleasant dreams and poor self-worth. "I felt ashamed and thought no one would ever want to marry me," she said. "I thank God that I did marry."

Once Esther left her parents' house and went to live with her supportive and kind husband, her incontinence became less frequent, although the nightmares and headaches remained. Often she found herself waking up after a nightmare with her bed wet. She also had sudden panic attacks, resulting in heart palpitations and shortness of breath. Esther had never told her husband about the history of her abuse for fear that he might not understand. Ashamed, she longed for help.

Her symptoms are common in post-traumatic stress disorder (PTSD), which occurs in people who have experienced trauma. Like her, many people struggle quietly with poor health resulting from abuse that may have started at a very young age. Our deepest and often most meaningful relationships, those behind the closed doors of our homes, can have a powerful influence on our health and well-being for life.

Physical Health Impact

Research has shown that supportive relationships strengthen the immune system and increase our ability to fight off illness and disease. One such study indicated that just three weekly visits by relatives and close friends improved the immune function in the seniors.[1] The other side of the coin is also true. Scientific investigation has documented that abusive relationships may damage our health. Exposure to physical, sexual, or emotional violence, or the ongoing stress related to abuse, has links to many health problems. Adverse childhood experiences appear to produce several physical health problems later in adulthood. The traumatic childhood events include "verbal, physical, or sexual abuse, as well as family dysfunction," such as witnessing adult domestic violence.[2] It is tragic that oftentimes those who have the strongest bonds to a human being—one's own family—can perpetrate such acts of violence. The home, which should be a little heaven on earth, a shelter and safe haven filled with warmth and love, can become a place of harm, danger, and fear behind closed doors.

Such an unhealthy environment becomes a source of chronic stress, possibly resulting in disease and even death. Adults who have experienced child abuse have up to a 60 percent higher risk for diabetes.[3] Studies of childhood neglect have also found an increased risk of diabetes.[4] The current pandemic of diabetes makes such facts both startling and worrying. Who would have thought that diabetes could have anything to do with the type of relationships we have at home? But such negative physical health effects go beyond that of diabetes or the immune system. Traumatic experiences in childhood appear to have a role in cancer, cardiovascular disease, obesity and being overweight, and early death.[5] The evidence strongly suggests that if excessive stress weakens the immune system in childhood and abuse damages the delicate mechanisms of the mind, multiple physical, mental, and emotional problems may surface later in life.

Mental and Public Health Impact

Unhealthy relationships at home actually cause changes in our brain. The parts of the brain particularly affected are those that play important roles in long- and short-term memory.[6] Additionally,

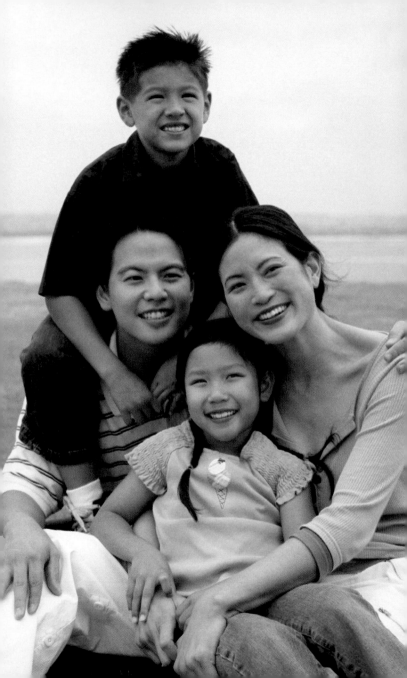

both children and adult victims of family violence often experience fear, shame, guilt, and stigma. Such negative emotions contribute to mental and emotional problems, including depression, bipolar disorder, and post-traumatic stress disorder in both men and women.[7]

Experiencing childhood maltreatment and poverty at an early age harms our immune system. The bodies of those who have endured such a background often show, when they become adults, an abnormal control of inflammation because of faulty immunity. They also have an increased risk for diabetes! Such immune system dysfunction appears not only in the case of child abuse, but also during adult conflict between spouses and companions, especially if it continues for some time.

Public Health Impact

Research has linked abuse and violence in all its forms not only to increased mortality but also to having a negative influence on the entire community. Globally, violence and abuse have become major problems.

The following statistics bring the health effects of violence and abuse into stark perspective: More than one in three female homicides worldwide occur at the hands of an intimate partner—often a spouse or companion.[8] Such violence commonly represents the end result of a long history of abusive relationships. Public health officials in the United States list violence among one of eight major priorities affecting the health of American citizens.

Protective Factors

Fortunately, even despite the many negative health outcomes among survivors of domestic violence, there is still hope! Not everyone who experiences abusive relationships will develop such health problems. Often described as resilience, many individuals manage to bounce back by employing effective coping mechanisms.

The good news for anyone affected by domestic violence is that such positive coping factors can help people to heal. They include cultivating wholesome emotions; learning to be flexible; developing a selfless concern for the well-being of others; having social support; and utilizing faith, religion, or spirituality.[9] In fact, studies suggest that gratitude, and forgiveness specifically,[10] can powerfully contribute to psychological resilience in the face of trauma and abuse.

Forgiveness or gratitude can be healing balms and protective factors that will enable us to deal with the disease that may result from abusive relationships. If someone has hurt you deeply and you fail to forgive them, you are allowing them to injure you a second time. An unforgiving spirit destroys our health and imprisons us in bitterness. It robs us of the joy God longs for us to have. Just as Jesus forgave those who crucified Him when they did not deserve it, so we can forgive those who have wounded us when they do not warrant it. Forgiving another does not mean that we condone their actions or justify what they did to us. Rather, forgiveness is releasing another from our condemnation when they do not deserve it, because Christ released us from His condemnation when we do not deserve it. As the apostle Paul so clearly states, "And be kind to one another, tenderhearted, forgiving one another, even as God in Christ forgave you" (Ephesians 4:32, NKJV).

One of the questions that people have when they experience the heart wrenching trauma of abusive relationships is, "Where is God in all of this?" Pain and injustice flood the globe. At times life is just plain unfair. We live in a world of good and evil, joy and sorrow, love and hate, health and sickness. Sometimes we bring heartache upon ourselves through our own poor choices, but there are plenty of times that we have done absolutely nothing wrong, and sorrow seems to stalk us. Trauma strikes. Tears flow. Tragedy overwhelms us. But in spite of all of life's injustice, God is still near. And He will never leave us or forsake us (Hebrews 13:5). Instead, if we will let Him, He strengthens and encourages. He still heals broken hearts, sets at liberty the captives, and delivers the oppressed (Luke 4:18).

Here is an eternal biblical truth that is life transformational: God is love (1 John 4:8). His actions toward us are always and only loving ones. He would never do anything to harm us. Whatever painful, traumatic childhood experiences you may have had in the past, God did not cause them, and you are certainly not responsible for them. They were the result of harmful, destructive choices made by someone else. Do you feel guilty for something you had absolutely no control over, or blame God for it? If there is an aching void in your heart because of childhood hurts, emotional betrayal, or physical or mental abuse, Jesus understands. He was Himself betrayed and beaten, ridiculed and rejected. People lied about and laughed at Him. His enemies cursed and crucified Him. But in spite of such horrible injustices, He never lost faith in His Father's love and care. Able to understand what you have gone through, He is near to heal your heart and give you new hope for living.

Have you ever wondered about the purpose of all human relationships? Why does God give us fathers, mothers, brothers, sisters, husbands, wives, sons, daughters, and friends? Each human relationship is part of God's plan to reveal a different aspect of His love. Throughout Scripture we find Him pictured as having the qualities of a strong caring Father, a tender pitiful mother, a loving husband, an affectionate wife, a protective big brother, a listening sister, and a faithful friend. God reveals His love through the prism of human relationships.

But what if one of those relationships gets fractured through no fault of our own? What if rather than revealing God's character qualities it reflects the brokenness of sin and the destructive nature of selfishness? When we learn to trust Him, God will bypass the relationship and fill our hearts with the love we should have received from the father, mother, sister, brother, husband, wife, or friend. Read the Bible passages below and let your heart rejoice that He can supply the deepest needs of your heart:

"As a father pities his children, so the Lord pities those who fear Him" (Psalm 103:13, NKJV).

"A father of the fatherless, a defender of widows, is God in His holy habitation" (Psalm 68:5, NKJV).

"Can a woman forget her nursing child, and not have compassion on the son of her womb? Surely they may forget, yet I will not forget you" (Isaiah 49:15, NKJV).

"For your Maker is your husband, the Lord of hosts is His name; and your redeemer is the Holy One of Israel; He is called the God of the whole earth" (Isaiah 54:5, NKJV).

"But there is a friend [Jesus] who sticks closer than a brother" (Proverbs 18:24, NKJV).

They are just a sampling of Bible passages that describe the close intimate relationship the Father, Son, and Holy Spirit desire to have with us. When behind closed doors our lives have been shattered, we can discover new hope in a God who will rebuild our lives and supply all that our hearts lack. Love flowing from the heart of an infinite God is healing love. In Him life is new. Through Him we can hope again, and because of Him, we can face the future with new joy.

[1] J. K. Kiecolt-Glaser et al., "Psychosocial Enhancement of Immunocompetence in a Geriatric Population," *Health Psychology* 4 (1985): 25-41.

[2] Centers for Disease Control and Prevention, "Adverse Childhood Experiences Reported by Adults," available at www.cdc.gov/mmwr/preview/mmwrhtml/mm5949a1.htm.

[3] V. J. Felitti et al., "Relationship of Childhood Abuse and Household Dysfunction to Many of the Leading Causes of Death in Adults," *American Journal of Preventive Medicine* 14 (1998): 245-258.

[4] R. D. Goodwin and M. B. Stein, "Association Between Childhood Trauma and Physical Disorders Among Adults in the United States," *Psychological Medicine* 34 (2004): 509-520.

[5] Centers for Disease Control and Prevention, "Adverse Childhood Experiences Reported by Adults."

[6] A. Danese and B. S. McEwen, "Adverse Childhood Experiences, Allostasis, Allostatic Load, and Age-related Disease," *Physiology & Behavior* 106 (2012): 29-39.

[7] J. McCauley et al., "Clinical Characteristics of Women With a History of Childhood Abuse: Unhealed Wounds," *JAMA* 277 (1997): 1362-1368.

[8] H. Stöckl et al., "The Global Prevalence of Intimate Partner Homicide: A Systematic Review," *The Lancet* 382 (2013): 859-865.

[9] K. Tusaie and J. Dyer, "Resilience: A Historical Review of the Construct," *Holistic Nursing Practice* 18 (2004): 3-8.

[10] A. J. Miller et al., "Gender and Forgiveness: A Meta-Analytic Review and Research Agenda," *Journal of Social and Clinical Psychology* 27 (2008): 843-876.

Chapter 6

You Are What You Think

A positive attitude is life-giving: nurture it.

Have you ever questioned why at times negative thoughts flood your mind? Have you ever wondered how to turn such negative thoughts into positive ones? Have you ever noticed the impact of how you think on what you do when faced with an important moral choice or ethical dilemma?

When a group of volunteers endured two sleepless nights, army researchers found that the lack of sleep hindered the participants' ability to make decisions in the face of emotionally charged moral dilemmas.[1] Perhaps even more significant, however, was that while some volunteers changed their views of what was morally acceptable as a result of sleep deprivation, it was not universally the case. Those who, at the beginning of the study, scored high on a measure known as "emotional intelligence" did not waver on what they found morally appropriate.

This study and many others help to confirm the eternal truth in Proverbs 23:7 that as a person "thinks in his heart, so is he" (NKJV). The way we reason shapes our responses to life. Our thoughts govern what we do. Our behavior often follows what is in our minds. We act out the images that we project on the screen of our conscience. It's clear that all of us must expect to face emotionally charged moral dilemmas at least sometime in our lives. And when we do, how will we respond? At such occasions emotional intelligence may be a plus.

What Is Emotional Intelligence?

Traditionally we have understood intelligence as the cognitive or mental capacity of a person, and the means employed to measure it is the IQ (intelligence quotient) test. Yet in 1983 developmental psychologist Howard Gardner proposed in *Frames of Mind* the theory of multiple intelligences. Instead of defining intelligence as a single logical ability, we should see it as a set of eight (later he included one more) clusters of skills: naturalist intelligence ("nature smart"), musical intelligence ("musical smart"), logical-mathematical intelligence ("number/reasoning smart"), interpersonal intelligence ("people smart"), bodily-kinesthetic intelligence ("body smart"), linguistic intelligence ("word smart"), intrapersonal intelligence ("self smart"), spatial intelligence ("picture smart"), and existential intelligence ("morality smart").[2]

Then in 1995 psychologist and science journalist Daniel Goleman launched an internationally best-selling book titled *Emotional Intelligence,* which popularized this kind of intelligence, normally defined as the sentimental capacity of the mind, or the ability to identify, assess, and control emotions. According to Goleman, emotional intelligence has five distinct aspects:[3]

(1) knowing our emotions
(2) managing our emotions
(3) recognizing emotions in others
(4) managing relationships with others
(5) motivating ourselves to achieve our goals

All of them are important, for we always need to decipher and manage emotions.

The Role of Emotional Intelligence

Emotional intelligence (EQ or EI) is not related merely to decision-making. Studies show that while the job a person gets after graduating from college might reflect their IQ, how far they advance in that job bears little relationship to it.[4] It's not even connected to their grades in school. Rather, it's related to their EQ. Our success and happiness in life are more closely associated with EQ than with any other form of intelligence.

A variety of scientific studies has shown that increasing a person's EQ will prevent or treat depression, phobias, obsessive-compulsive disorder, post-traumatic stress disorder, anorexia, bulimia, and addictions such as alcoholism.[5] The 12-step program of Alcoholics Anonymous, for example, has achieved remarkable success, but it is four times more successful if combined with a program to enhance emotional intelligence.

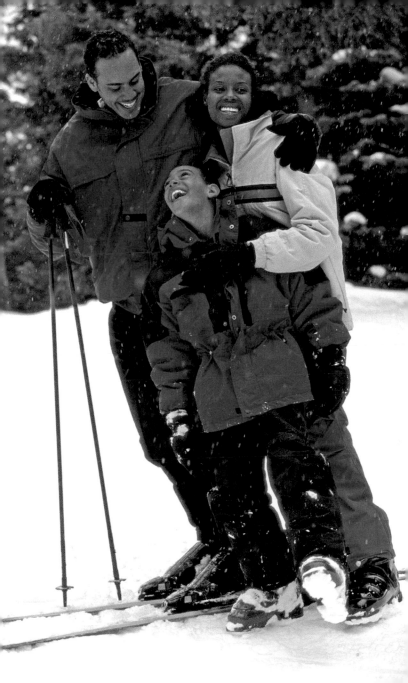

What about persons who don't necessarily have an addiction or a specific disease?

Enhancing EQ will help those individuals to think more clearly and communicate more effectively. It fosters unity in group settings, reduces polarizing statements, and promotes a happier life.

Influences on Emotional Intelligence

Researchers have done extensive studies during the past decade on what can influence EQ. Our genetic makeup, childhood experiences, and current level of emotional support all play a role. So does what we eat.

Bonnie Beezhold has shown that a plant-based diet is associated with healthier mood states in both men and women.[6] Switching to a vegetarian diet will reduce levels of stress, anxiety, and depression, apparently because plant foods don't have arachidonic acid, an inflammatory fat present largely in meat and fish.

Our activities have an impact on both our IQ and EQ The more entertainment television watched, the lower the creativity and one's grades.[7] In addition, a lack of emotional control—including an increase in violent and sexual crimes—results.[8] Entertainment Internet, videos, and video games also have an adverse effect. As the apostle Paul stated: "By beholding we become changed" (see 2 Corinthians 3:18).

The most important influence on EQ, however, is what we believe. Our beliefs—that is, our evaluations of events, the way we think about problems, our silent (or sometimes not-so-silent) self-talk—largely shape our emotions. Thus our beliefs have much more to do with how we feel than what is actually happening in our lives.

Let's take an example from the Bible. The local authorities arrested and cruelly beat Silas and Paul without a fair trial. They then tossed the two onto a rough dirt floor and fastened their feet in stocks (Acts 16:22-24). But they sang praises to God. Why? Because their thoughts were more powerful than what was actually taking place in their life. We can learn and develop emotional intelligence by espousing several principles. Let's illustrate three of them through biblical examples.

The Case of Saul

King Saul was tall, handsome (1 Samuel 9:1, 2), and wealthy. Such characteristics, however, have very little to do with emotional intelligence.

Negative thoughts began to develop in his mind that represented irrational, twisted thinking. We know of at least three causes of his mental turmoil. The first was *cognitive distortion of magnification and minimization*—in other words, magnifying things that are not important, and minimizing things that are truly significant.

How did Saul minimize? When confronted with his guilt, he blamed others and justified himself (1 Samuel 15:20, 21). "Why don't you just talk about what I did right?" he complained to the prophet Samuel, who had confronted him. "You're focusing on things I didn't do right, which, by the way, aren't such a big deal." He did not learn from his mistakes.

Saul also *dwelt on the unfairness of his life*. As a result of his guilt, he received a sentence, and Saul thought that the punishment outweighed the crime. But did it? After all, God had issued the verdict Himself. We must acknowledge that not everyone always gets treated fairly, but even in such adverse situations, dwelling upon that unfairness will inevitably cause significant emotional problems.

The third aspect of Saul's distorted thinking, connected to magnification, was an *inordinate self-esteem* (verses 16-19). We can also call it an inflated pride that was easily wounded—in his case, by the people's, and especially the women's, obvious preference for another leader (1 Samuel 18:6-9).

If we do not find ourselves constantly elated by applause, if we have humility and not a distorted magnification of self, we are less likely to become seriously depressed by censure or disappointment. That doesn't mean that we should have a low sense of self-worth. A Christian recognizes that Christ would have died for just one soul, making each of us of infinite value. But when we think that we're more important than the person sitting next to us, for whom Christ also died, we have crossed the line into arrogance and pride.

Although Saul was a man with wonderful potential, he lived a selfish life, never completely trusting and obeying God, and never giving up his pride for more than a few days. Finally, under tremendous stress and with his enemies closing in, his sad life ended in suicide.

The Case of Solomon

A second cognitive distortion is *emotional reasoning*, which goes like this: I feel like a failure, therefore I am a failure. I feel overwhelmed and helpless, thus my problems are impossible to solve. I feel as if I'm on top of the world, therefore I'm invincible. I'm angry at you, and that proves you've been cruel and insensitive to me. Such emotional reasoning often results in a cycle of addiction.

In the biblical book of Ecclesiastes Solomon wrote, "I said to myself, 'Come now, I will test you with pleasure to find out what is good.' But that also proved to be meaningless. . . . I denied myself nothing my eyes desired; I refused my heart no pleasure" (Ecclesiastes 2:1-10, NIV).

If someone is having fun, Solomon said, I want to do what they're doing. The interesting thing is that even though we actually have more "fun things" to do today than ever before, depression is epidemic in our society. Thus if pleasurable things could prevent or treat depression, we should see the lowest levels of depression. But that's not the case.

Most of the "fun things" in which people in our society participate spike the dopamine levels in our brains, creating a sense of pleasure, but they also result in a subsequent dramatic drop far below the normal level afterward. Furthermore, the more we do such things, the less they spike. Pretty soon, when we engage in our addiction of choice, it takes us barely up to neutral. In the in-between times, however, we feel a deep, overwhelming sense of sadness.

Solomon also wrote, "I hated life . . . for all is vanity and vexation of spirit. Therefore I went about to cause my heart to despair" (verses 17-20). He had the most money, the most beautiful houses and gardens, and the most beautiful women. His contemporaries thought he should be the happiest of persons. But his selfish gratification did not bring happiness. "By his own bitter experience, Solomon learned the emptiness of a life that seeks in earthly things its highest good."[9]

Eventually Solomon turned his life around. And if his dissipated life could be redirected, there's hope for every one of us.

Jonatan Martensson points to a solution for emotional reasoning. "Feelings are much like waves," he observes. "We can't stop them from coming, but we can choose which one to surf." And we can select them on the basis of what is true and in harmony with God's plan for our life.

The Case of Elijah

Elijah "went a day's journey into the wilderness, and came and sat down under a juniper tree: and he requested for himself that he might die; and said, It is enough; now, O Lord, take away my life, for I am no better than my fathers!" (1 Kings 19:4). The Old Testament prophet didn't have a sense of inflated pride, nor did he engage in a self-indulgent lifestyle. He lived a simple life. Yet he suffered from significant depression.

A man who had always followed God's will, Elijah had just experienced God's miraculous intervention on Mount Carmel. Yet within a day someone informed him that he was about to lose his life, and he panicked. Did Elijah have reason to fear Jezebel? Yes, because she had killed all the other prophets of the Lord. But instead of depending upon God's protection, he turned and ran. Forty days later he was so depressed that he wanted to die.

God had to put Elijah on a depression-recovery program. Like many depressed people, the prophet wanted to be in the dark—in the cave. God had to send an earthquake and a whirlwind to get him out of the cave and into the light. After those things, however, the Lord turned to what was most important to Elijah's recovery. He provided cognitive behavioral therapy to correct the prophet's distorted thoughts.

Elijah's distortion was *overgeneralization.* "I am the only one who has not bowed down to Baal," he said. The Lord let him get by with it the first time. But then the prophet repeated it, and God couldn't let him continue any longer in his self-destructive overgeneralization. "Elijah," the Lord said, "there are 7,000 others who haven't bowed to Baal."

To help Elijah overcome his depression, God gave him a set of specific tasks (verses 15, 16). The prophet followed through on what the Lord asked him to do, and he not only recovered, but God took Elijah to heaven without him seeing death (2 Kings 2:11).

Set Free

If the thoughts are wrong, the feelings will be wrong—and thoughts and feelings combined make up the personal character. But the good news is that reconstructing our thinking *will* change us. The Bible says, "Be transformed by the renewing of your mind" (Romans 12:2, NIV). We not only have to recognize distorted thoughts, but must correct them and replace them with true and accurate ones that find their source in God.

How then can we safeguard and improve our emotional intelligence? By eating healthy foods; getting adequate sleep; avoiding bad entertainment on the Internet, television, and movies; and rejecting cognitive distortions: self-magnification, emotion-based reasoning, overgeneralization, and so forth.[10] We must fill our minds with accurate and true thoughts, ones derived from an understanding of God's plan for our lives. Then, Christ says, "you shall know the truth, and the truth shall make you free" (John 8:32, NKJV).

The way to get rid of negative thoughts is by replacing them with positive ones. Self-defeating, depressing thoughts will rush into our minds. But at those times, the counsel of the apostle Paul is extremely helpful: "Set your mind on things above, not on things on earth. For you died, and your life is hidden with Christ in God. When Christ who is our life appears, you will also appear with Him in glory" (Colossians 3:2-4, NKJV). Notice this divine instruction carefully. First it counsels us to "set our mind on things above." We might rephrase it this way: "Choose to fill your mind with the reality of divine truth. Do not allow the distortions the devil brings to you to shape your thinking."

"Setting our minds on things above" makes a major difference in our thought processes for two significant reasons. First, we sense anew that "our life is hidden with Christ in God." In Him we are affirmed and accepted. And in Him we are safe and secure. He is our refuge and strength. On the cross Jesus triumphed over all of the forces of evil. His victory is ours (Colossians 2:15). Nothing can rip us out of His hands (John 10:27, 28). Nothing can separate us from His love (Romans 8:35-39). And nothing can rob us of our deep inner peace and joy if by faith we daily grasp the reality that our real life is in the protection of Jesus and God.

Second, "setting our minds on things above" is powerfully life-transformational because "when Christ who is our life appears" at the Second Coming, we will join Him in glory. This is hope and encouragement beyond anything that might trouble and harass us. Jesus is coming again to take us home. One day sorrow, suffering, disease, and depression will be over. Oppression and injustice will fade into the eternal past. In Christ, through Christ, and because of Christ, we can think positive, hopeful, joyous thoughts today and throughout all eternity.

---

[1] W.D.S. Killgore et al., "The Effects of 53 Hours of Sleep Deprivation on Moral Judgment," *Sleep* 30 (2007): 345-352.

[2] See Howard Gardner, *Frames of Mind: The Theory of Multiple Intelligences* (New York: Basic Books, 2003).

[3] See Daniel Goleman, *Emotional Intelligence: Why It Can Matter More Than IQ* (New York: Bantam Books, 1995).

[4] M. D. Aydin et al., "The Impact of IQ and EQ on Pre-eminent Achievement in Organizations: Implications for the Hiring Decisions of HRM Specialists," *International Journal of Human Resource Management* 16 (2005): 701-719.

[5] L. M. Ito et al., "Cognitive-behavioral Therapy in Social Phobia," *Revista Brasileira de Psiquiatria* 30 (2008): S96-101; T. D. Borkovec and E. Costello, "Efficacy of Applied Relaxation and Cognitive-Behavioral Therapy in the Treatment of Generalized Anxiety Disorder," *Journal of Consulting and Clinical Psychology* 61 (1993): 611-619; G. A. Fava et al., "Six-year Outcome of Cognitive Behavior Therapy for Prevention of Recurrent Depression," *American Journal of Psychiatry* 161 (2004): 1872-1876.

[6] B. L. Beezhold, C. S. Johnston, and D. R. Daigle, "Vegetarian Diets Are Associated With Healthy Mood States: A Cross-sectional Study in Seventh Day Adventist Adults," *Nutrition Journal* 9 (2010), available at www.nutritionj.com/content/pdf/1475-2891-9-26.pdf.

[7] I. Sharif and J. D. Sargent, "Association Between Television, Movie, and Video Game Exposure and School Performance," *Pediatrics* 118 (2006): e1061-70.

[8] L. R. Huesmann et al., "Longitudinal Relations Between Children's Exposure to TV Violence and Their Aggressive and Violent Behavior in Young Adulthood: 1977-1992," *Developmental Psychology* 39 (2003): 201-221; B. J. Bushman and C. A. Anderson, "Media Violence and the American Public: Scientific Facts Versus Media Misinformation," *American Psychologist* 56 (2001): 477-489.

[9] Ellen G. White, *Prophets and Kings* (Mountain View, Calif.: Pacific Press Pub. Assn., 1917), p. 76.

[10] Neil Nedley, *The Lost Art of Thinking: How to Improve Emotional Intelligence and Achieve Peak Mental Performance* (Ardmore, Okla.: Nedley Pub., 2011).

Chapter 7

HOPE BEYOND DEPRESSION

There is a better day coming: anticipate it.

Depression is a global problem that can affect anyone anywhere. Statistics reveal that more than 350 million people of all ages suffer from it. The leading cause of disability worldwide, it is a major part of the global burden of disease. Those who study the patterns of disease predict that such figures will only increase in the future.

The World Health Organization describes depression as "a common mental disorder," characterized by sadness, loss of interest or pleasure, feelings of guilt or low self-worth, disturbed sleep or appetite, feelings of tiredness, and poor concentration."[1] At its worst, depression can lead to suicide. An estimated 1 million people die depression-related deaths each year. This is even more disturbing when we realize that a number of positive principles and effective treatments can make a major difference for people dealing with depression.

Even a better standard of living does not ensure happiness. "Based on detailed interviews with over 89,000 people, [study] results showed that 15 percent of the population from high-income countries, compared to 11 percent for low/middle-income countries, were likely to get depression over their lifetime, with 5.5 percent having had depression in the last year."[2] As we see, money is not a solution to disappointment, discouragement, and despair.

The same research shows that women are "twice as likely to suffer depression as men, and the loss of a partner, whether from death, divorce or separation, was a main contributing factor."[3] The cause of depression is not the same for everyone. For some, it is a genetic problem that affects the balance of chemicals (neurotransmitters) in the brain. For others, a stressful life event, such as the death of a loved one, losing a job, a divorce, or some equally distressing life event, may trigger it. In many cases depression occurs as a result of the combination of both the chemical imbalance and a triggering event. Whatever the cause, whether it is a chemical upset in the brain or the heartache of some major life event, depression can harm a person's life and needs effective solutions.

A Serious Condition

Depression can be very disabling. Millions of people live in the dark shadow of sadness, gloom, and hopelessness, and often struggle with feelings of inadequacy and worthlessness. While there are degrees of depression—and we all experience minor versions of it—almost 22 women out of every 100 will have an episode or more of major depression during their lifetime. That is almost double the chance of such an event occurring in men. Approximately 13 out of every 100 men during their lifetime cope with some form of depression. Children up to the age of 10 may also experience depression, though the gender difference is not apparent until the reproductive years during and after adolescence. Once they pass menopause, though, women become less prone to depression.

Multiple factors make women more susceptible to stress- induced depression than men. They also are about four times more prone to seasonal-affective depression than men. It is the form of depression that occurs in areas where winter daylight hours are very short. People wake up and go to work in the dark and return home in darkness, and have little exposure to sunlight. Yet another factor that may influence the onset of depression is the hormonal fluctuations of the reproductive years. They may well affect neurotransmitters in the brain, increasing vulnerability to depression.

Women in many cultures do not enjoy equal status with men, something that could also play a role in depression. The demands placed upon women to produce children or to regulate family size mean that they often carry disproportionate responsibilities and accountability for reproductive function. Infertility or a miscarriage may get viewed as a failure to fulfill their role. Oral contraceptives may carry a potential for depression in susceptible women. Hormonal factors may play a cyclical (occurring monthly) role or during the postpartum state following childbirth. Whatever the causes, women with depression need and deserve serious and compassionate care.

The symptoms of depression vary from person to person. Persistent tiredness and loss of energy are common complaints among those suffering from it. Depressed individuals may suffer from loss of concentration and become indecisive. Feelings of guilt and low self-worth often persist for weeks and even months at a time. Some may experience difficulty in sleeping or, on the other hand, sleep more than normal. Many find themselves waking up early. Persons suffering from depression tend to lose interest in daily activities. They may struggle with recurring thoughts of death and suicide. Changes in eating patterns may cause either weight loss or weight gain (a change of more than 5 percent of body weight in a month). In severe cases, individuals with depression lose interest in eating and no longer find pleasure in any of life's activities, including social relationships.

Society needs to recognize that the major depressive disorders are as much a disease as the more physical ones, such as diabetes or hepatitis. Ill-advised comments such as "pull yourself together" or "get a grip" reflect either a lack of knowledge or, even more sadly, the ignorance of the one making them. Such statements may cause further pain, heartache, and a worsening of the depression.

Treatment of Depression

A person with a major depressive illness will need professional help. It is dangerous and ill-advised for even well-meaning but untrained health enthusiasts to try to interfere in the life of a person struggling with the condition.

There exist a number of approaches to the treatment of major depression. Anyone who has symptoms of depression must seek the aid of an informed and qualified health professional. Careful evaluation will help to determine the precise form of treatment needed. Severe cases may call for hospital admission. Along with medication, such programs will provide counseling and a helpful approach such as cognitive behavioral therapy. Patients may often take medication for a number of months and, sometimes, require repeated treatments.

Minor depression in men and women will often respond to programs of exercise. The Harvard Medical School reports some encouraging news about dealing with depression: A review of studies stretching back to 1981 concluded that "regular exercise can improve mood in people with mild to moderate depression—and may even play a supporting role in treating severe depression."

The report further states that "study published in *Archives of Internal Medicine* assigned 156 depressed patients to an aerobic exercise program, the SSRI sertraline (Zoloft [a kind of antidepressant]), or both. At the 16-week mark 60 to 70 percent of the people in all three groups no longer had major depression. In fact, group scores on two rating scales of depression were essentially the same." "A study published in 2005 . . . found that walking fast for about 35 minutes a day five times a week or 60 minutes a day three times a week significantly improved symptoms in people with mild to moderate depression."[4]

If you are feeling a little down, get out, take a walk, and breathe deeply. While you do so, meditate on God's goodness and ask Him to fill your mind with positive thoughts.

Another factor in dealing with depression involves the food we eat. Changes in them may also ease some of the situation. The Mayo Clinic reports that diet may contribute to depression: "Some preliminary research suggests that having a poor diet can make you more vulnerable to depression. Researchers in Britain looked at depression and diet in more than 3,000 middle-aged office workers over the course of five years. They found that people who ate a junk food diet—one that was high in processed meat, chocolates, sweet desserts, fried food, refined cereals, and high-fat dairy products—were more likely to report symptoms of depression."[5]

In other words, when you eat your veggies, you are benefitting your brain as well as your body. Now, don't misunderstand us—we are not suggesting that consuming a carrot a day will keep you singing all the time. Depression is a complex subject, but a healthy diet is part of an overall wellness program that will assist in reducing the problem.

Some general health habits can also be effective:

- Eat healthfully of a well-balanced plant-based diet.
- Have regular sleep and rest routines.
- Exercise regularly in the outdoors.
- Cultivate meaningful relationships with family and friends.
- Trust in the power and grace of our loving heavenly Father.

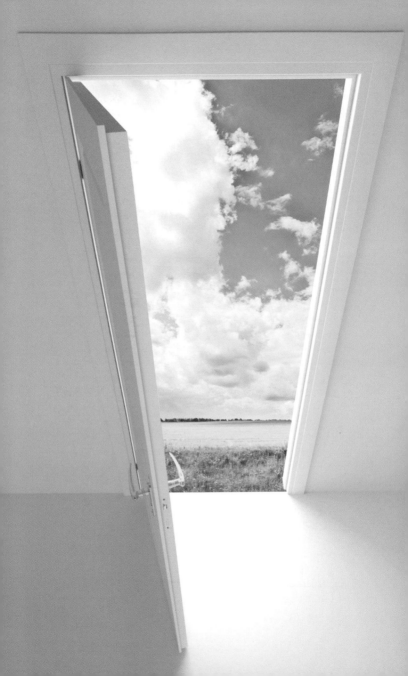

- Change your pattern of thought, trying to focus your mind on possibilities and positive things.
- Seek professional help if you experience symptoms of depression for prolonged periods, and then follow the prescribed treatment of qualified health personnel.

One of the strongest antidotes for depression is social support. Warm, loving relationships, close friendships, and strong family ties make all the difference. If you are feeling down, confide in a friend, share your burden with someone you can trust. You do not need to bear it alone. In fact, Jesus Himself invites us to bring our heaviest burdens to Him. He says, "Come to Me, all you who labor and are heavy laden, and I will give you rest" (Matthew 11:28, NKJV).

When dealing with depression, proper stress management can be helpful, as well as a balanced spiritual relationship with God. That was the experience of an ancient prophet in biblical times. We already talked about him in the previous chapter, but let us revisit his story and see what else it can teach us.

Stress constantly filled Elijah's day, such as when he confronted the idolatrous prophets of the pagan god Baal on Mount Carmel. It had not rained for three and a half years. Crops had failed and famine stalked the land. Elijah raised a challenge: If the God of heaven was supreme and all powerful, let Him send rain. But if Baal was more powerful, let him answer the prayers of his prophets and pour down showers. After all, that was what his worshippers claimed he had charge of. The tension mounted, and the pressure grew. The prophets of Baal wailed their meaningless prayers, and nothing happened. Then Elijah petitioned heaven, and the rain came. The prophet of God witnessed a miracle, and he was elated. But his mountaintop experience would soon turn to despair.

Jezebel, King Ahab's wife, now threatened Elijah's life. Exhausted and fearful, God's prophet fled. The further he journeyed, the more depressed he became. Despondency settled over him like a dark cloud. Confused and discouraged, he had no desire to live. Scripture records the story this way: "But he himself went a day's journey into the wilderness, and came and sat down under a broom tree. And he prayed that he might die, and said, 'It is enough! Now, Lord, take my life, for I am no better than my fathers' " (1 Kings 19:4, NKJV). Elijah became so depressed that life did not appear worth living any longer.

Commenting on the incident, one Christian writer adds: "Into the experience of all there come times of keen disappointment and utter discouragement—days when sorrow is the portion, and it is hard to believe that God is still the kind benefactor of His earthborn children; days when troubles harass the soul, till death seems preferable to life. It is then that many lose their hold on God and are brought into the slavery of doubt, the bondage of unbelief. Could we at such times discern with spiritual insight the meaning of God's providences we should see angels seeking to save us from ourselves, striving to plant our feet upon a foundation more firm than the everlasting hills, and new faith, new life, would spring into being."[6]

At this critical point in Elijah's life God provided food and water for the prophet, urged him to get some rest, and encouraged him with the assurance that He was still with him. Eventually Elijah left his dungeon of despair and once again rejoiced in the sunlight of the Lord's joyous presence.

In many respects, Elijah's story is that of each one of us. Everyone at some point suffers with depression resulting from life's challenging events. At such times we can count on God's help.

A High Note

So let's end the chapter on a high note. Cynthia (pseudonym), a professional colleague of one of the authors of this book, experienced prolonged and deep depression. But in time, as she followed some of the counsels given here, she broke free from the despair that enslaved her. Here is her counsel to anyone experiencing a similar situation: "If you are depressed for a prolonged period of time, get help. Don't rule out medication. Medication can break down the wall of darkness that surrounds you, and this breakthrough will give you the strength you need to make lifestyle changes that could assist your recovery. Find a good, highly recommended doctor. Share your struggle with someone else, and ask that person to pray for you."

"If your depression is a life struggle, feed on the Word of God," she advises. "Read and memorize 'joy' texts, such as Nehemiah 8:10,

Psalms 34, 40, and 66, and the book of Philippians. Begin a 'joy journal' in which you give God thanks for five things each night before you go to sleep. Feed your mind with good things. Highlight texts in your Bible that talk of joy, rejoicing, gladness, and praise, so that you can claim those texts each day." Finally, she always likes to quote a phrase written by a Hebrew poet: "Because You have been my help, therefore in the shadow of Your wings I will rejoice" (Psalm 63:7, NKJV).

Remember this eternal truth: it is a law of the mind that it gradually adapts itself to the subjects you allow it to dwell on. Fill your mind with positive thoughts. Meditate upon God's Word. Claim His promises as your own. Believe that Jesus, the light of the world, will illuminate your darkness. Do not accept lies about you. A valuable child of God, you mean more to Him than you will ever know. Understanding our worth in His sight and His care for us will help us to thrive!

[1] World Health Organization, "Depression," Fact Sheet No. 369, available at www.who.int/mediacentre/factsheets/fs369/en/index.html.

[2] BioMed Central, "Global Depression Statistics," available at www.sciencedaily.com / releases/2011/07/110725202240.htm.

[3] *Ibid.*

[4] Harvard Health Publications, *Understanding Depression* (Boston: Harvard Medical School, 2008), available at www.hrccatalog.hrrh.on.ca/InmagicGenie/DocumentFolder/understanding%20depression.pdf.

[5] Mayo Clinic, "Diseases and Conditions: Can a Junk Food Diet Increase Your Risk of Depression?" available at www.mayoclinic.org/diseases-conditions/depression/expert-answers/depression-and-diet/faq-20058241.

[6] E. G. White, *Prophets and Kings,* p. 162.

Chapter 8

BREAKING FREE

Balance is the pathway to success: seek it.

It was a scene of heartrending pain: crying children and a frustrated mother, obviously emotional and angry. "This is the last straw," she said to herself. "We can't take it anymore!" Sam, the alcoholic father and husband, had lost yet another job.

A pleasant, soft-spoken man, he generally was a kind father and considerate husband—except when under the influence of alcohol. Well liked and welcomed into the sporting circles of his town, he could always be counted on to participate in the celebrations at the clubhouse or pub after a golf game or other sporting event. As his addiction to alcohol cost him one job after another, however, he lost not only his financial security but also the many friends with whom he had played, drunk, and fraternized during the "better" times.

He had a problem not only with alcohol—he also smoked cigarettes. Not even the discovery of cancer of the larynx had motivated him to stop smoking for more than a few months. Life-threatening diagnoses such as heart attack and cancer often lead only to short-term lifestyle changes. The sobering reality is that it requires something more to effect meaningful and long-term transformations in our established behavior.

Sam's sad story bears witness to such a pattern, described best in his own words during his numerous but short-lived periods of recovery: "I can control tobacco and alcohol; they are not my master!" The sad reality is that they *were* his master, and he was, in fact, their slave.

His love affair with alcohol affected many others, especially those in his family. Two of his four children also became alcoholics. Truly the wise man was right when in Proverbs 23:29-32 he declared:

"Who has woe? Who has sorrow? Who has contentions? Who has complaints? Who has wounds without cause? Who has redness of eyes? Those who linger long at the wine, those who go in search of mixed wine. Do not look at the wine when it is red, when it sparkles in the cup, when it swirls around smoothly; at the last it bites like a serpent and stings like a viper" (NKJV). In other words, whether you realize it or not, alcohol is a deadly substance. Sam discovered its terrible truth too late.

Perhaps you believe that moderate drinking is good for your health. But do you know that there isn't a safe level of alcohol consumption that will not lead to an increase in breast cancer among women and colon cancer among men? Also there are the problems of addiction, accidents, domestic violence, and other health and societal issues associated with alcohol use. If alcohol is part of your lifestyle, know that life can be much better without it.

How Big Is the Alcohol Problem?

According to the "Global Status Report on Alcohol and Health" released by the World Health Organization in Geneva in February 2011:[1]

- Approximately 2.5 million people die from alcohol-related causes each year.
- Fifty-five percent of adults have consumed it.
- Almost 4 percent of all deaths worldwide are related to alcohol through injuries, cancer, cardiovascular diseases, and liver cirrhosis.
- Globally, 6.2 percent of male deaths involve alcohol.

The World Health Organization report also revealed that worldwide in 2005, 6.13 liters of pure alcohol were consumed per person age 15 years or older. The amount appeared to be stable in the Americas and the European, Eastern Mediterranean, and Western Pacific regions. However, the researchers noted marked rises in Africa and Southeast Asia. Health risk increases even more with binge drinking or when people drink solely to get drunk. Definitions of binge drinking vary, but in the United States health officials consider more than five consecutive drinks for a male and more than four for a female as binge drinking. The practice of binge drinking is exploding in many parts of the world.

Alcohol consumption leads to tens of thousands of preventable deaths each year. "In the European Union [EU], alcohol accounts for about 120,000 premature deaths per year: 1 in 7 in men and 1 in 13 in women," says another report of the World Health Organization.[2] Such worrying facts place alcohol alongside tobacco as one of the world's leading preventable causes of death and disability.[3] No ordinary commodity, alcohol is very dangerous.

Alcohol Addiction

Of every 100 people who drink alcohol, 13 will develop alcoholism during their lifetimes. If there's a first-degree relative (e.g., father, mother, uncle, aunt, grandparent) who has suffered from alcohol dependence, the likelihood doubles. But should experimentation with alcohol begin under the age of 14 years, the chance of becoming addicted increases to 40 percent-plus![4]

We need to educate children about the dangers of alcohol from an early age. Parents and others must foster healthy relationships and connectedness from an early age. Such social support develops resilience and promotes healthful choices. An additional layer of protection for both young and old is a vital, personal faith in God.

Why is faith so important when dealing with addictions? Because of two very significant reasons. First, an understanding that our bodies are not fun houses, but the temple of the living God makes all the difference. The Christ who both created us and redeemed us longs to live in us through His Holy Spirit. The apostle Paul's words echo down the corridors of time: "Or do you not know that your body is the temple of the Holy Spirit who is in you, whom you have from God, and you are not your own? For you were bought at a price; therefore glorify God in your body and in your spirit which are God's" (1 Corinthians 6:19, 20, NKJV).

The second reason faith makes so much difference in our ability to overcome destructive habits is that when we choose to surrender our weak, wavering wills to God, He strengthens us to be able to

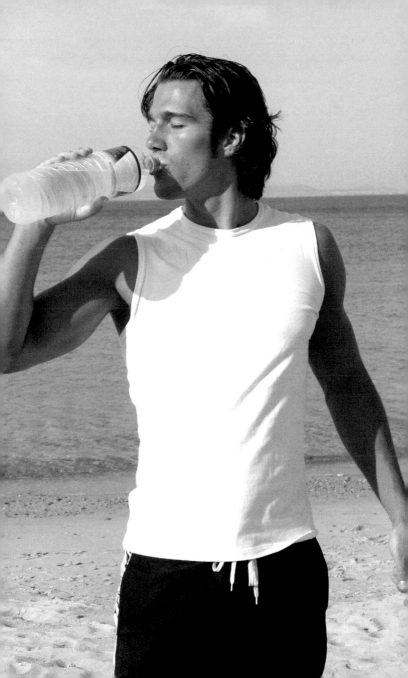

overcome destructive lifestyle habits. The apostle John states it succinctly: "For whatever is born of God overcomes the world. And this is the victory that has overcome the world—our faith" (1 John 5:4, NKJV). Our loving heavenly Father desires that each one of us live a life free from crippling addictions that predispose us to life-threatening diseases such as heart disease and cancer.

Alcohol and Cancer

Cancer is one of the leading causes of death worldwide. Researchers in the European Union, where cancer has become the second-most-common cause of death (with about 2.5 million cancer deaths per year), estimate that alcohol consumption directly causes 10 percent of cancers in men and 3 percent of those in women. Avoiding alcohol could prevent approximately 30 percent of total cancers in the European Union.[5] Worldwide, we find strong evidence that alcohol triggers breast cancer in women and colon cancer in both men and women. There appears no safe limit/dose of alcohol that will avoid its carcinogenic (cancer-causing) effect. It is, therefore, clearly dangerous for anyone to recommend alcohol use to enhance health, as some are doing for possible cardiac benefits.

Alcohol and Society

It's well known that alcohol use lies behind accidents of all kinds, such as road fatalities, as well as domestic violence, murder, rape, and other criminal activities. Alcohol is also the leading cause of preventable mental retardation in the world. It easily crosses the placenta and damages the developing brain of the unborn baby. As a result, there is no safe level of alcohol consumption during pregnancy.

Alcohol and Heart Health

For the past 30 years some have promoted alcohol as "heart healthy" and protective against coronary artery disease. Much has appeared in popular and scientific publications on the subject. But the many contradictory results of the various studies may be for a wide variety of reasons. Prominent researchers have suggested that some or all of the apparent cardiac protective effect of moderate drinking may be the result of other factors.[6] Differences in health status, education, and socioeconomic status of the individuals studied have added even more confusion in interpreting the data. For example, a number of the subjects included in the nondrinking group had been drinkers prior to the studies being done and had stopped using alcohol for health reasons.[7] A growing number of researchers attribute the better heart health outcomes among the moderate drinkers not to alcohol, but to their average health status and healthful lifestyle in other behaviors, such as exercise and a diet that were superior to that of the nondrinkers studied.[8]

Taking into account all the definite health risks related to alcohol, it doesn't make sense to promote its use for heart health, especially when other proven and safe ways to prevent heart disease exist, such as daily exercise and a healthful diet.

Killer Tobacco

Another killer is tobacco. Every day more than 1 billion people smoke or chew tobacco, and 15,000 die daily from tobacco-related diseases.[9] Most of those deaths could be avoided if people did not smoke, as well as still more if we eradicated secondhand smoke. The bottom line is: If you smoke, you put yourself at risk.

Tobacco is a lethal and freely available poison marketed in various forms. It's smoked, chewed, inhaled, used electronically, and even dissolved in water (*shisha*). All forms are harmful, substantially increasing the risk of disease and even death. Tobacco kills up to half its users!

- Tobacco contributes to the deaths of nearly 6 million people each year. Six hundred thousand of them are nonsmokers exposed to secondhand smoke.
- Nearly 80 percent of the world's 1 billion smokers live in low- and middle-income countries.
- Consumption of tobacco products continues to increase globally.
- Approximately one person dies every six seconds as a result of tobacco-related causes.

- Up to half of current users will eventually die of a tobacco-related disease.

Tobacco is a gradual killer with a lag of several years between starting to use tobacco and when the user's health deteriorates. It's one of the most significant public health threats the world has ever faced, not only killing the user but often negatively affecting the health of, or even killing, those exposed to secondhand tobacco smoke. Tobacco smoke contains more than 2,000 chemicals and substances. At least 250 of them are known to be harmful, and more than 50 cause cancer.

Secondhand smoke by definition is the smoke that fills restaurants, offices, homes, and any enclosed space in which tobacco products burn, including cigarettes, cigars, pipes, *bidis,* and water pipes (*shisha*). With no safe level of exposure, it's a proven cause of cardiovascular and respiratory disease in adults, including lung cancer and coronary heart disease. In babies it can cause sudden infant death syndrome. Children in contact with secondhand smoke have more upper- and lower-respiratory infections.

Furthermore, tobacco is a "gateway drug."[10] Those who use it place themselves at risk of using and becoming addicted to other drugs, such as marijuana, methamphetamine, cocaine, and heroin.

Both alcohol and tobacco are extremely dangerous. Scientific evidence and public health statistics show them to be leading killers in the world today. It's a personal choice whether to use tobacco, alcohol, or other harmful, health-destroying substances, but our choices have consequences.

The facts certainly speak for themselves. We were created for something better than to experience preventable diseases as a result of our poor decisions. Remember that it is never too late to begin making positive lifestyle choices, and when we do, God comes immediately to our aid to empower our decisions. What we could never accomplish on our own we can through His strength.

Enemy Number One

As far back as 1971 then-president Richard Nixon stated that "America's public enemy number one in the United States is drug abuse. In order to fight and defeat this enemy, it is necessary to wage a new, all-out offensive."[11] If it was true at that time, it is much more so today, and the same reality applies also to other countries.

Because of its illegal nature, we can have no precise statistics about the size of the illicit drug industry. Experts have estimated it at $300 billion, $400 billion, and even $1 trillion per year.[12] In 2010 United Nations Office on Drugs and Crime calculated that between 153 million and 300 million people ages 15 to 64 took drugs during the previous year, with a higher prevalence of cannabis (marijuana) followed by amphetamine-type stimulants. As a rule, the use of illicit drugs by males far exceeds that by females, who, more often resort more to tranquillizers and sedatives.[13]

It has been estimated that only 20 percent of problem drug users receive treatment for their dependence. The tragedies resulting from such dangerous consumption are staggering. The number of deaths as a consequence of drugs has been calculated to be between 99,000 and 253,000. In some countries great numbers of murders are drug-related. For example, the Mexican government estimates that 90 percent of the killings in the country have connections with drugs. While that may be an extreme case, it still tells us much about the malignant potential of illicit drugs.[14]

The impact of drug use on one's health is beyond description. Many think about it only when a celebrity such as Philip Seymour Hoffman dies. According to the medical examiner, the Oscar-winning actor was killed "by a toxic mix of drugs." However, numerous ordinary people get sick and die every day as a result of drug abuse.

Drugs affect almost every organ of the body. They can weaken the immune system, increasing susceptibility to infections; cause cardiovascular problems, including abnormal heart rate, heart attacks, and infections of the blood vessels and heart valves; provoke nausea, vomiting, and abdominal pain; damage the liver; trigger stroke; alter brain chemistry, leading to substance dependency; do permanent brain damage; affect memory, attention, and decision-making; induce paranoia, aggressiveness, hallucinations, depression, and addiction; and "may pose various risks for pregnant women and their babies."[15]

Fortunately the drug users and their families don't need to face the challenge alone. Many treatment centers and support services can help. Narcotics Anonymous is one of them. Its vision is that "every addict in the world has the chance to experience our message in his or her own language and culture and find the opportunity for a new way of life."[16] With human and divine help, victory is possible.

True Balance in Living

You may be struggling with the shackles of addiction to alcohol, tobacco, drugs, overwork, pornography, media addiction, or just living an unbalanced life. Few feelings can match the sheer desperation of attempting to give up something and failing, and then continuing to try and still failing. Habits form easily, but are difficult to break. In fact, sheer grit and willpower ("won't power," if you will!) are not enough to gain victory over enslaving habits and addictions. We need help.

A great missionary and writer, the apostle Paul, described our source of strength as a power outside ourselves. Fortunately, he also shared the secret of such power and success: "I can do all this through him who gives me strength" (Philippians 4:13, NIV). He also adds, "No temptation has overtaken you except such as is common to man; but God is faithful, who will not allow you to be tempted beyond what you are able, but with the temptation will make the way of escape, that you may be able to bear it" (1 Corinthians 10:13, NKJV). Whatever challenge you face, others have too. You are not alone in your struggles. And whatever we may face, God has already made a way of escape. In His strength you find can a fulfilling life that is physically, mentally, emotionally, and spiritually balanced.

Even the most strong-willed among us cannot achieve this true balance without a strong reliance on the power of our gracious and all-powerful God who not only created us but is able to sustain us and strengthen our will and ability to make wise choices. He then encourages us further in our quest for wholeness, even in our brokenness: "Whether you eat or drink or whatever you do, do it all for the glory of God" (1 Corinthians 10:31, NIV). Avoiding harmful, addictive, and destructive habits and practices then becomes a spiritually motivated decision made out of gratitude for the amazing and wonderful blessings and privilege of the gift of life.

It's encouraging to remember that help is never far away. Our gracious heavenly Father stands ready to guide our choices, ensuring a sustained and successful true balance in life. This applies as well to the prevention of, and victory over, destructive habits. Ask God to help you right now! You will not only survive, but also thrive!

[1] Available online at www.who.int/substance_abuse/publications/global_alcohol_report/en.

[2] "Status Report on Alcohol and Health in 35 European Countries 2013," available online at www.euro.who.int/en/publications/abstracts/status-report-on-alcohol-and-health-in-35-european-countries 2013.

[3] Thomas Babor et al., *Alcohol: No Ordinary Commodity,* 2nd ed. (New York: Oxford University Press, 2010), p. 70.

[4] Richard K. Ries et al., *Principles of Addiction Medicine,* 4th ed. (Philadelphia: Lippincott Williams and Wilkins, 2009).

[5] EuroCare, European Alcohol Policy Alliance, "Alcohol and Cancer—the Forgotten Link," available online at www.eurocare.org/library/latest_news/alcohol_and_cancer_the_forgotten_link.

[6] Timothy S. Naimi et al., "Cardiovascular Risk Factors and Confounders Among Non-drinking and Moderate-Drinking U.S. Adults," *American Journal of Preventive Medicine* 28 (2005): 369-373.

[7] Kaye Middleton Fillmore et al., "Moderate Alcohol Use and Reduced Mortality Risk: Systematic Error in Prospective Studies," *Addiction Research and Theory* 14 (2006): 101-132.

[8] B. Hansel et al., "Relationship Between Alcohol Intake, Health and Social Status, and Cardiovascular Risk Factors in the Urban Paris-Ile-de-FranceCohort," *European Journal of Clinical Nutrition* 64 (2010): 561-568.

[9] Robert Beaglehole et al., "Priority Actions for the Noncommunicable Disease Crisis," *Lancet* 377 (2011): 1438-1447.

[10] World Health Organization, "Tobacco," Fact Sheet No. 339; available online at www.who.int/mediacentre/factsheets/fs339/en/index.html. See also Omar Sharey et al., *The Tobacco Atlas,* 3rd ed. (Atlanta: American Cancer Society, 2009).

[11] Richard Nixon, "Remarks About an Intensified Program for Drug Abuse Prevention and Control," June 17, 1971. Available online by John T. Woolley and Gerhard Peters, The American Presidency Project, at www.presidency.ucsb.edu/ws/?pid=3047. For a chronology of America's drug war, see www.pbs.org/wgbh/pages/frontline/shows/drugs/cron/.

[12] See www.unodc.org/pdf/WDR_2005/volume_1_chap2.pdf.

[13] Data available at www.unodc.org/documents/data-and-analysis/WDR2012/WDR_2012_Chapter1.pdf.

[14] *Ibid.*

[15] Gateway Foundation, "Effects of Drug Abuse and Addiction," available online at http://recovergateway.org/resources/individuals/drug-addiction-effects/.

[16] Visit the Web site www.na.org/.

Chapter 9

BOUNCING BACK

A challenge creates a champion: embrace it.

During the past few decades researchers have begun to focus on the question Why do some youth who live in very high-risk environments *not* engage in dangerous behaviors? They conclude it all revolves around the term *resilience.*

Resilience is the ability to continue to function healthfully in spite of personal adversity, the various stresses of life, or even a destructive environment. Such resilience appears to develop as a result of a wide variety of social support. Despite severe hardships and the presence of at-risk factors, resilient individuals develop coping skills that enable them to succeed in life. They have a strong self-concept, a belief in God, and a positive attitude toward the world around them. Driven by a definite sense of purpose for their lives, they see life's obstacles as challenges that they can overcome. Above all, resiliency seems to be all about hope and a positive belief that there is life beyond today's obstacles.

Living in a High-Risk World

Although families, churches, and communities all seek to protect them, today's youth still live in a world filled with great risk. Very explicit sexual material awaits them with just a click on the Internet, and the majority of youth report that access to alcohol, marijuana, cocaine, and amphetamines is relatively easy—even in what many might consider as safe, wholesome environments. Therefore, it is important that we identify those factors that enable some young people to be successful despite the dangerous world they live in. Once we know that, we can help other youth to employ those same survival strategies.

The concept of resilience is vital today. If we can't make the home and social environments ideal; if we can't get the drugs off the street or remove violence from television, movies, and video games; and if we can't eliminate the harmful material from the Internet, then how can we assist children who grow up exposed to all these influences to remain healthy and succeed in life? What can we as individuals, as a church, or as a community do to help youth become resilient?

The first important thing to remember is that resilience appears to result from *supportive relationships!* In addition, resilient youth often have the ability to use their religious faith to maintain a positive vision of a meaningful life.[1]

The Role of Relationships

Valuable, sincere, and enduring positive relationships are key to developing resilient young people. Supportive older adults or mentors, including parents, teachers, clergy, or any responsible adult, all play a major role developing resilience. Relationships with individuals who provide care, warmth, and unconditional love appear to provide young people with a sense that they can overcome whatever odds life may throw at them. Such relationships can instill youngsters with a sense of self-worth that enables them to cope more successfully. One particular study found that "resilient youngsters all had at least one person in their lives that accepted them unconditionally."[2]

Resilience and Family Dinners

One effective and yet quite simple strategy that builds resilience is eating together as a family. A number of recent studies report that family dinners contribute to a lowering of risky and addictive behaviors in adolescents and young adults. Researchers have identified family dinnertimes as a protective factor against such risk behaviors as alcohol and substance use, smoking, early sexual activity, eating disorders, and delinquency.

Family dinners may reduce the likelihood of youth becoming the victims of violence.[3]

Also they appear to create better social and mental stability. Children and teenagers who share family dinners and spend time with their parents develop higher self-esteem, experience less depression, and have lower rates of suicide or thoughts of suicide.

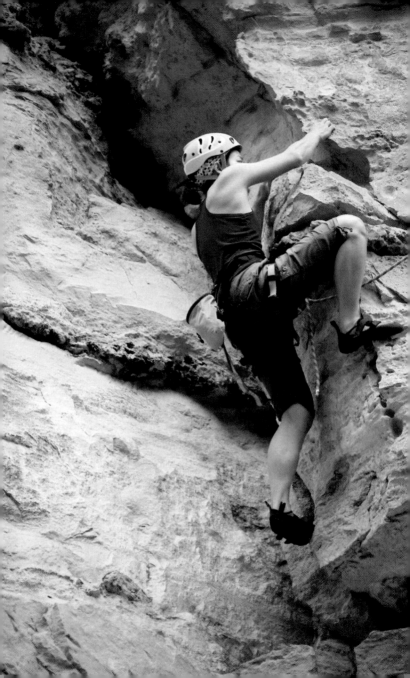

In addition, family meals also contribute to healthier eating habits and nutrition. Most important, they provide an ideal time to nurture spiritual values and a belief in God. Research on the subject of resilience has found that a belief in God plays a major role in future success and the ability to overcome difficult life circumstances.

Eating together as a family is a positive influence because of the family connectedness. Family bonding is one of the strongest factors that produce resilience. Thus family meals create an environment in which the family can communicate with one another, build lasting bonds between parents and their children, discuss problems and solutions, and cultivate a sense of stability. Parents can use family mealtimes to get to know and hear about their children's friends and others with whom they interact outside the home. Also mealtime offers opportunities to plan future events and activities that further bond the family together.

Job demands, as well as electronic devices, interfere with the sense of connectedness that should occur at mealtimes. It's crucial that parents turn off the TV and not allow the use of electronic devices during mealtimes. Nothing should interfere with the bonding that happens at family dinners. It is encouraging that youth actually enjoy the socializing of family meals.

Resilience and Service

Community service is another activity that promotes resilience among young people. It is a concept firmly established in Scripture. Jesus taught us much about serving others. In Matthew 25:31-46 He reveals that His people *serve* others by meeting their needs—such as feeding the hungry and clothing the naked. We are to show caring compassion and give assistance to all His people. Such practical activity provides us with still another method for protecting our kids from high-risk behaviors while, at the same time, encouraging their faith and belief. Thus we serve others not just by giving money, but also—together with our youth—by personal and practical assistance.

We can define service activities as any assistance that benefits those living in our local community. It is imperative to feed, clothe, and protect people. Beyond that, we can support, visit, aid, and comfort others who are in a position of need for any reason. But some may ask, "What does service have to do with kids and high-risk behaviors?"

First of all, it changes young people's lives. Through service they are much more likely to engage in healthy pro-social behaviors. Some years ago senator John Glenn, then chair of the National Commission on Service Learning and a famous astronaut, indicated that more than 80 percent of schools that had service as part of the school curriculums reported that the majority of participating students improved their grades.[4] Is it not interesting that by following Jesus' Matthew 25 directive, youth benefit personally? Involvement in service also strongly relates to a lower rate of high-risk behaviors and a significantly lower use of alcohol.[5]

Faith-based groups can often play a leading role in community service. They can organize service opportunities and provide responsible adult leadership. And it's the presence of responsible, caring adults that makes the difference. During service activities adults can show they really care about the lives of a young person, serve as role models, and share core spiritual and life values that relate to success. Adult mentoring in service activities can help overcome the negative effects of a difficult home environment.

In order for communities and young people to live life to the fullest, we must each do our part to develop resilient youngsters free of risky behaviors. Nurturing caring relationships, sharing the value of family meals, and implementing community service programs that encourage youth participation help to achieve this goal. It will make all the difference in the lives of our young people.

[1] T. P. Hebert, "Portraits of Resilience: The Urban Life Experience of Gifted Latino Young Men," *Roeper Review* 19 (1996): 82-90.

[2] R. Brooks, "Children at Risk: Fostering Resilience and Hope," *American Journal of Orthopsychiatry* 64 (1994): 545-553.

[3] D. C. McBride et al., "Family Dinners and Victimization," presented at the American Society of Criminology, Chicago, Illinois, November 2012.

[4] John Glenn, "The Benefits of Service-Learning," *Harvard Education Letter*, January/February 2001, available online at http://hepg.org/hel/article/150.

[5] G. L. Hopkins et al., "Service Learning and Community Service: An Essential Part of True Education," *Journal of Adventist Education*, May/June 2009, pp. 20-25.

Chapter 10

REST FOR OUR RESTLESSNESS

Rest is the remedy for fatigue: cherish it.

Tales come from eighteenth- and nineteenth-century England about how factory managers stole time from their workers. The managers would simply push the hands of the clocks back as the day progressed, forcing the unfortunate employees to work longer hours without extra pay. Another ploy involved having the minute hand move in three-minute intervals during the lunch hour instead of one, thus shortening the break. Such practices robbed the workers of the one commodity that we can never make up, and that is time.

We may lose money in the stock market or in other bad investments, but we can sometimes get it back. Or if we lose our health, we may sometimes regain it through proper medical attention, diet, and exercise. But time lost or stolen—whether one minute, one day, one week, whatever—is gone forever. In the movie *In Time* (2011) society controls the aging process in order to avoid overpopulation. Having much money, rich individuals can purchase a longer life span than those who are poor. However, what is possible in fiction is impossible in real life. Nobody can buy time.

The clock ticks onward regardless of what we do. From every direction forces work to take our time from us just as surely as a pickpocket will our wallets. Faster phones, faster electronic tablets, faster Internet connections, and faster computers have not, it seems, resulted in more time for us. On the contrary, it's one of the sad facts of the modern world that the faster we do things, the less time we have for ourselves. And although lack of time is a great ailment of modern life, a powerful antidote to our modern dilemma actually comes from antiquity. It's called Sabbath, and it is, along with proper sleep, one of the best ways to find rest for human restlessness.

Refuge

In parts of the world in which hurricanes, tornadoes, and tsunamis occur, people build shelters. Such shelters exist for one reason: to give people refuge from storms, particularly tornadoes. But there's a problem: we have to get to the shelter. If we are not near one and the storm strikes, we can be without refuge. No such shelter ever seeks us out—we have to go to it.

God, however, has created one that, instead of us having to rush to it, it comes to us! At 1,000 miles an hour (the speed of the earth's rotation), the Sabbath circles the globe. Arriving on one sundown, leaving on the next, the seventh-day Sabbath washes over the planet, bringing with it to our homes and lives a refuge from the world's ceaseless demands upon us and upon our time. This refuge, this rest, is so important that God offers it to us once a week, without exception. Our Sabbath rest is a symbol of our trust in our loving Creator, who cares for us more than we can imagine. On Sabbath we find shelter and protection from life's cares, anxieties, and problems.

The Sabbath symbolizes our rest in the One who loves us more than we can imagine. Abraham Heschel, a prominent Jewish author, described the Sabbath as a "palace in time."[1] Once a week God's heavenly palace descends from heaven to earth for 24 hours and our Creator opens to us the glory of His presence. Free from earth's perplexities and the worrisome burdens of daily living, we are shut in with Him in our Sabbath sanctuary of refuge. God not only invites us into His Sabbath rest, but commands us to worship and to cease from our work. He knows that a life of incessant hurry and constant work will break down our life forces, weaken our immune systems, and so absorb our focus that we would forget about Him. Along with the commandments against killing, stealing, and adultery, we find the commandment to rest. That tells us how important it is for our general well-being. But the rest that our Lord is speaking about is much more than a physical one, although it surely includes sleep. It is the total rest of mind, body, and spirit in the context of His love and care for us.

Sleep and the Sabbath Rest

Without question, among all the things the Sabbath is about and all the things it brings to us, rest is central. Even the name itself in Hebrew, *Shabbat,* comes from a verb that means "to cease, to rest." Yet no matter how crucial the Sabbath rest can be, in and of itself it's just not enough. Resting one day a week, however beneficial spiritually, mentally, and physically it is to us, would be insufficient without another kind of rest—that of sleep.

God doesn't come right out and command us to get enough sleep, as He does for us with our Sabbath rest. He doesn't need to because our bodies themselves, if we will listen to them, give us the commands. It's up to us whether we'll heed them or not. In a sense, as the Sabbath always comes to us, sleep does the same.

Of course, just as violating God's commands brings negative consequences, ignoring what our body tells us will as well. In 2011 a Chinese man died after a three-day marathon he spent in front of the computer in a cybercafé almost without eating and drinking. Two years later, in December 2013, Mira Diran, a young employee of the advertising agency Young & Rubicam in Indonesia, worked continuously for three days. She used energy drinks to keep awake. But the price she paid for her extravagant dedication was death.

It's amazing how bleak and gloomy the world can seem when seen through eyes drooping from sleep-deprived exhaustion. On the other hand, the sense of rebirth and renewal after a long night of deep sleep is totally refreshing. After all, if God created human beings to work (Genesis 2:15), He also created them to rest. And between the rest of the Sabbath and that of sleep, and the blessing of balanced, productive work, we can enjoy optimal physical, spiritual, and mental well-being. Sabbath and sleep are the true rest for human restlessness.

Sleep

Scientific research is clear: as human beings we need sleep. Without enough of it, we cannot function properly. Everyone, whether they will admit it or not, knows how important sleep is. Yet despite years of study, it still remains a mystery. Exactly what it is, what it does, and why it affects our bodies and minds the way it does are questions that still need many answers. We do know that sleep is

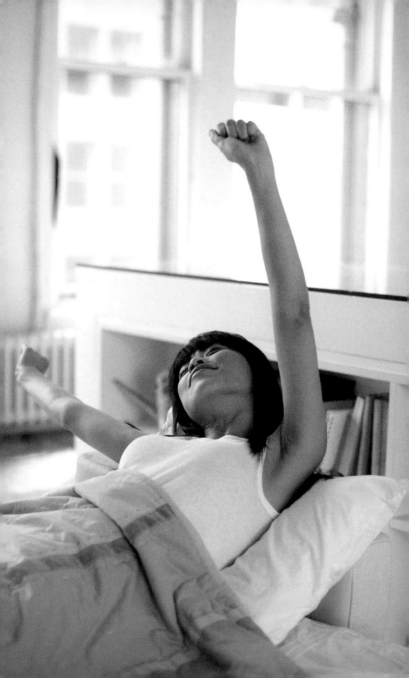

essential to health and well-being. While it does not guarantee that you won't get sick, the lack of it means that sooner or later you will.

How much sleep is enough? The answer varies, because people, their health, their work habits, their age, and their metabolism vary. For practical purposes, most people need about eight hours of sleep a night (some studies put the range between seven and nine hours). It is the optimal amount necessary to experience sleep's full benefits. Besides just helping us feel rested and better emotionally and physically, sleep helps fight off infection, prevents diabetes, and reduces the risk of heart disease, obesity, and high blood pressure.

"Sleep health is a particular concern for individuals with chronic disabilities and disorders such as arthritis, kidney disease, pain, human immunodeficiency virus (HIV), epilepsy, Parkinson's disease, and depression. Among older adults, the cognitive and medical consequences of untreated sleep disorders decrease health-related quality of life, contribute to functional limitations and loss of independence, and are associated with an increased risk of death from any cause."[2]

Sleepless Around the World

Despite laborsaving devices, jet travel, and high-speed Internet, we are not getting enough sleep. You would think that with everything being done faster, we'd have more time to rest and relax. But many around the world are sleeping less than the recommended seven to nine hours. In addition, an increasing number of people have sleep problems, with many millions suffering from some type of chronic sleep disorder.

Lack of sleep leads to decreased performance during the day. Reducing sleep by even one and a half hours, even for just one night, results in a drop of daytime alertness by as much as 32 percent. Furthermore, lack of sleep weakens memory and cognitive skills. And who hasn't experienced the added stress caused by someone's crankiness or irritability from not enough sleep? Workplace accidents are twice as likely to happen in cases in which one of the workers didn't get sufficient sleep. The National Highway Traffic Safety Administration (NHTSA) estimates that each year drowsy driving leads to at least 100,000 automobile crashes, 71,000 injuries, and

1,550 fatalities just in the United States. Because problems caused by lack of sleep affect those around us as well, it becomes, therefore, our responsibility to get adequate sleep and rest.

Tips for Better Sleeping

Although some people have serious sleep issues that require medical attention, here are a few simple hints that can help most of us have the restful sleep we need:

- Take your sleep seriously. Be intentional about getting adequate sleep and rest each night.
- Develop regular sleep patterns. Our bodies work on rhythms, so try to go to bed at the same time every night and get up at the same time, even on weekends.
- Regular physical exercise (the amount your doctor recommends for you) can be very beneficial in helping you get a good night's sleep. When you exercise, your body burns up energy, and sleep is the best way (along with eating proper food) to restore it. "The sleep of a labouring man is sweet" (Ecclesiastes 5:12).
- Do not to go to sleep on a full stomach. Develop the routine of a light evening meal and avoid food for at least two hours prior to going to bed.
- Avoid caffeinated beverages, as caffeine is a stimulant and may keep one awake.
- Avoid stressful situations before going to sleep. Take the TV out of the bedroom permanently. Resolve family disagreements during daylight hours, not at bedtime.
- Focus on spiritual things and claim God's promises about trusting and resting in Him. "Rest in the Lord, and wait patiently for him" (Psalm 37:7). Many people find it extremely beneficial to read from Psalms before they go to sleep each evening. The psalms tend to bring calm to our lives and a peace to our souls. They relax the mind and prepare it for sleep.

Weekly Rest

Sleep is not the only component of our overall need of rest. As we have seen, God commands the weekly Sabbath rest, because He knew that, unless ordered to do it, we wouldn't take the necessary rest. If people, so driven by the desire to get ahead, to earn more money, to learn more, don't allow themselves even enough physical sleep, who would keep the Sabbath as well? Yet, like all God's commandments, the weekly Sabbath rest is for our own good. He told the children of Israel: "Keep the commandments of the Lord, and his statutes, which I command thee this day for thy good" (Deuteronomy 10:13). And one of those commandments "for thy good" was to rest on the Sabbath day.

God instituted the Sabbath as part of the original Creation Week. That is, even before any of the other Ten Commandments existed, the sanctity of the Sabbath rest already did: "Thus the heavens and the earth were finished, and all the host of them. And on the seventh day God ended his work which he had made; and he rested on the seventh day from all his work which he had made. And God blessed the seventh day, and sanctified it: because that in it he had rested from all his work which God created and made" (Genesis 2:1-3).

The Lord did not originally intend the blessing of the Sabbath just for any one people. He created the day of rest for all humanity, because all people have their origins in the Lord. "God saw that a Sabbath was essential for man, even in Paradise. He needed to lay aside his own interests and pursuits for one day of the seven, that he might more fully contemplate the works of God and meditate upon His power and goodness. He needed a Sabbath to remind him more vividly of God and to awaken gratitude because all that he enjoyed and possessed came from the beneficent hand of the Creator."[3]

Achieving true rest demands much more than merely the physical act of sleeping. Finding rest for our restless minds and bodies requires something beyond putting our heads on our pillows in mindless slumber. It is entering into heaven's Sabbath rest—that is, setting aside the seventh-day Sabbath as the day that God blessed and then stepping away from all we do and spending time with Him and contemplating what He has done for us. Those who have experienced the peace, the serenity, the joy that comes from anticipating the Sabbath rest and partaking of it week after week, know just how physically, spiritually, and mentally beneficial it can be for work-weary souls.

Choose to Rest

If we aren't careful, the demands on our time can dominate us even to the detriment of our physical, mental, and spiritual health. God has given us two powerful ways to break those vicious cycles of time, two ways to find rest for our restlessness: sleep and the Sabbath. We ourselves can choose to find the rest both of sleep and of the Sabbath. But most of all, heaven longs for us to discover the joy of resting totally, fully, and securely in Jesus, thus experiencing His true rest both now and throughout all eternity.

[1] Abraham Joshua Heschel, *The Sabbath* (New York: Farrar, Straus and Giroux, 1979).
[2] HealthPeople.gov, "Sleep Health," available at http://healthypeople.gov/2020/topics objectives2020/overview.aspx?topicid=38.
[3] E. G. White, *Patriarchs and Prophets,* p. 48.

Chapter 11

THE HEALING POWER OF FAITH

Faith is a great health restorer: receive it.

For decades researchers have examined the relationship between faith and health. Today we have a mounting body of evidence that faith does make a difference in our total well-being. Faith in a personal God who loves us and only has our best good in mind has a positive impact on both our physical and emotional health. What we believe about God affects every area of our lives. Our spiritual beliefs and practices make a difference in our total well-being. Thus our spiritual lives play a far greater role in determining our overall health than we previously understood.

Although the research is continuing, we clearly realize that faith does matter. Here's a sampling of what researchers have discovered that a dose of spirituality can do for you:

1. Stress: A comprehensive study conducted in Alameda County, California, followed the lifestyle practices of nearly 7,000 Californians. It revealed that West Coast worshippers who participate in church-sponsored activities are markedly less stressed about finances, health, and other daily concerns than nonspiritual individuals.[1]

2. Blood pressure: Senior citizens in a Duke University study who attended religious services, prayed, or read the Bible regularly had lower blood pressure than those who did not follow such practices.[2]

3. Recovery: A Duke University study discovered that devout patients recovering from major surgery spent an average of 11 days in the hospital compared with nonreligious patients, who spent 25 days in the hospital.[3]

4. Immunity: Research on 1,700 adults found that those who attend religious services were less likely to have elevated levels of interleukin-6, an immune substance prevalent in people with chronic diseases.[4]

5. Lifestyle: A review of several studies suggests that spirituality has links with lower suicide rates, less alcohol and drug abuse, less criminal behavior, fewer divorces, and higher marital satisfaction.[5]

6. Depression: Women with "pious" moms are 60 percent less likely to be depressed than those whose mothers aren't so reverent, according to a Columbia University study. Daughters belonging to the same religious denomination as do their mothers are even less likely (71 percent) to suffer the blues while sons were 84 percent less likely.[6]

Wholeness in Brokenness

Faith and spirituality, however, are not all that one needs to have perfect health. Since the arrival of sin, we all to some degree suffer physically, mentally, and spiritually, regardless of how much faith in God we have.

In the Bible Job, a man of great faith, endured devastating physical ailments. Paul pleaded three times for God to remove his particular thorn in the flesh, but instead of physical healing of his "brokenness," he received a special kind of wholeness: "My grace is sufficient for you," the Lord told him, "for My power is made perfect in weakness" (2 Corinthians 12:9, NIV). No wonder Paul could say, "For when I am weak, then I am strong" (verse 10, NIV).

Such encouragement is particularly meaningful to those who, despite faith, prayer, and medical intervention, still suffer from chronic diseases.

Faith Makes a Difference, but Questions Remain

The research is very convincing: faith does make a difference in our physical as well as our spiritual lives. But significant questions still remain. If we have enough faith, can we live as we please and still be healthy? Does faith give us license to violate the laws of health and still expect to live longer?

Assuming that if you have enough faith your lifestyle choices will make little difference is a misguided presumption that may quickly lead you to end up in the hospital. The idea that faith is some type of magic cure that makes medical professionals unnecessary is a major misunderstanding. Some people believe that if you go to the doctor for a medical problem, you lack faith. They fail to understand that the same God who can heal directly more often guides the skilled medical professionals to accomplish it. *All* healing comes ultimately from God. He is the Great Healer. But *how* He heals and *whom* He uses to accomplish the healing process is up to Him.

Faith Defined and Applied

Let's explore genuine biblical faith, as well as consider its source and results. To understand the meaning of faith, we'll begin with Hebrews 11:1: "Now faith is the substance of things hoped for, the evidence of things not seen" (NKJV).

What is faith, then? It is the substance. The Latin word "substance" comes from two other words: "sub" and "stance." "Sub," of course, means "under." We have words such as "submarine," a boat that travels under the sea, and "subterranean," something under the earth. The word "stance" refers to the essence of a thing. The substance is the thing that stands under everything else in your life, supporting, sustaining, and securing it. Faith is the very foundation of our existence.

Standing beneath everything else, it supports all our hopes and sustains us as we grapple with the perplexing questions of life. The essence of a vibrant spiritual life, faith keeps it from crumbling. Abel, Enoch, Noah, Abraham, Jacob, Moses, Joseph, and the other heroes of Hebrews 11 all had one thing in common: faith, a faith that sustained and supported them throughout their lives.

Faith is a relationship with God as a well-known friend, which leads us to do whatever He asks and accept whatever He allows with the absolute assurance that He only wants the best for our lives. It believes that God will strengthen us to triumph over every difficulty and overcome every obstacle until the day we receive our final reward in His eternal kingdom. Thus faith leads you to trust God as someone who loves you, knows what is good for you, and is interested in your happiness.

Energizing our entire being, faith lifts our spirits, encourages our hearts, renews our hope, and changes our vision from what is to what can be. Believing God's promises, it receives His gifts before they even materialize.

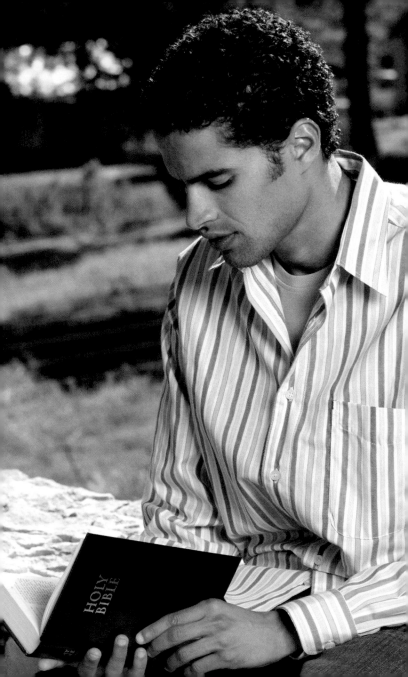

Heaven's Hall of Fame

In Hebrews 11 God lists the heroes of faith down through the ages. Their names hang high in heaven's "Hall of Fame." It's surprising that the first example of faith that He gives in Hebrews 11 is of someone who dies without any miraculous deliverance. "By faith Abel offered to God a more excellent sacrifice than Cain, through which he obtained witness that he was righteous, God testifying of his gifts; and through it he being dead still speaks" (Hebrews 11:4, NKJV).

According to the Bible, Abel was a righteous individual. But what was the result of his faith? It got him killed. If he hadn't had faith, he would have lived. Cain did not have faith and lived, while Abel who did have faith, died. That may seem strange to some people who have a mistaken understanding of genuine faith, such as those who believe that if you have enough faith you will always be healed.

Now, let's consider Enoch, the next in Scripture's royal line of faith: "By faith Enoch was translated that he should not see death; and was not found, because God had translated him: for before his translation he had this testimony that he pleased God" (verse 5).

If Enoch didn't have faith, he would have died. But he did have faith, so he lived. Yet Abel had the same quality of faith and perished. One thing does not puzzle us, however. Each of the worthies of faith in Hebrews 11 teaches us how to trust God. Enoch trusts Him in life, and Abel does so in death.

Now let's look at Noah's example: "By faith Noah being divinely warned of things not yet seen, moved with godly fear, and prepared an ark for the saving of His household" (verse 7, NKJV). His faith led him to do just what God said, even though to the majority of people in his day it must have seemed ridiculous. Obediently Noah followed God's instructions. Trusting Him, he remained where he was for 120 years building an ark despite the fact that there was no rain. Now, that's faith.

Abraham's experience is just the opposite: "By faith Abraham obeyed when he was called to go out to the place which he would afterward receive as an inheritance. And he went out, not knowing where he was going" (verse 8, NKJV). His faith led him to leave the security of his homeland and venture out into the unknown.

What contrasts! Abel died by faith, and Enoch survived by it. Noah stayed by faith, and Abraham ventured out because of it.

Sarah conceived a child by faith when she was 90 years old, and years later Abraham took her son, Isaac, to Mount Moriah at God's command to sacrifice him. There the Lord honored Abraham's faith and delivered the lad. The same God who asked the parents to believe He would give them a child now asked them to believe when He commanded them to sacrifice him. Of course, God miraculously provided deliverance for Isaac, foreshadowing Jesus' sacrifice and miraculous deliverance of each one of us from the jaws of sin and death.

Here's another contrast found in Hebrews 11. Joseph was faithful to God in spite of the difficult circumstances of his life. As the result of his faithfulness, God honored him. He lived as a witness of the true God amid the wealth and opulence of Egypt. But Moses had the opposite experience. The Lord led him out of Egypt to wander in the wilderness in total dependence on Him. Moses chose to "suffer affliction with the people of God than to enjoy the pleasures of sin, esteeming the reproach of Christ greater riches than the treasures in Egypt; for he looked to the reward" (verses 25, 26, NKJV). Joseph had faith and remained in Egypt, while Moses had faith and God told him to leave Egypt. Through faith Joseph became rich, but Moses became poor.

Faith is seeking God's will for my life, whether it's in death as with Abel or in life as with Enoch. Whether it's staying like Noah or going like Abraham, or whether it's living in the luxury of Egypt like Joseph or being a homeless wanderer in the desert like Moses, faith is always an abiding trust in God.

What circumstance do you find yourself in today? Is it facing a life-threatening illness or enjoying good health? Are you perfectly content in your home or anticipating a move and dreading it? prospering financially or struggling to pay your mortgage? enjoying a great marriage or finding yourself in a stressful, strained relationship? Do you feel very close to God or distant from Him? Faith, however, is not dependent on our feelings or situations.

Each of the heroes in God's Hall of Fame in Hebrews 11 experienced different circumstances in their lives. Faith does not hinge on what's going on around us but has everything to do with what's going on inside us. Each of the worthies of faith in Hebrews 11 had one common thread running through their lives: they trusted God.

Faith is trusting God for:

- strength in our weakness
- hope in our depression
- guidance in our doubt
- joy in our sorrow
- peace in our anxiety
- wisdom in our ignorance
- courage in our fear

Not knowing defeat or understanding the word "impossible," faith is filled with courage. Trusting God in all life's circumstances, faith can remain positive whatever happens, because it trusts in the one who knows no defeat. It's that trusting attitude of faith that causes the brain to release positive chemical endorphins, which strengthen the immune system and bring health to our bodies.

Faith's Source

Faith is not some kind of hyped-up positive thinking or self-induced warm feeling. It is not our ability to make ourselves believe something. Hebrews 11:6 describes the source of all faith: "But without faith it is impossible to please Him, for he who comes to God must believe that He is, and that He is a rewarder of those who diligently seek Him" (NKJV).

The source of all faith is an all-powerful, all-knowing, all-loving God. A trusting relationship with the Lord begins with the realization that He loves us and desires only good for us.

Our attitude also plays a significant part in our well-being. It's not just our lifestyle that determines our health. Human emotions also have a significant impact. A study reported by researchers from the University of Kansas found that positive emotions are critical to maintaining good physical health, especially for those deeply impoverished. In other words, if you want to be healthy, you need a positive attitude, particularly if you're enmeshed in difficult circumstances. The study showed that positive emotions such as happiness and contentment are unmistakably linked to better health, even when taking into account a lack of basic needs.

Carol Ryff, psychology professor at the University of Wisconsin–Madison, noted: "There is a science that is emerging that says a positive attitude isn't just a state of mind. It also has linkages to what's going on in the brain and in the body." Ryff has shown that individuals with higher levels of well-being have lower cardiovascular risk, lower levels of stress hormones, and lower levels of inflammation.[7]

God is the source of all positive emotions, and faith taps into those emotions and releases healing power into the body. Faith is trusting God in every circumstance of life, and no other attitude is as life-giving or health-restoring.

Increasing Our Faith

What do you do when your faith is weak? Perhaps you may agree that faith is life-giving, yet feel that you don't have much faith. We have good news for you. You have more faith than you realize. The problem is not that you don't have any faith—it's that you haven't exercised what you have.

In Romans 12:3 Paul says: "As God has dealt to each one a measure of faith" (NKJV). When we make a conscious choice to reach out to our all-loving, all-powerful God and trust Him, He places within our hearts a measure of faith.

Faith is a gift that God gives us. The more we exercise that gift, the more it will grow. As we learn to trust Him amid the trials and challenges we face in life, our faith increases. Sometimes our moments of greatest desperation are those of our greatest growth in faith.

We can also expand our faith as we meditate upon God's Word. As the truths of the Bible fill our minds, our faith increases rapidly. The Scriptures affirm this divine reality in Paul's letter to the Romans: "So then faith comes by hearing, and hearing by the word of God" (Romans 10:17).

The more we saturate our minds with Scripture, the greater our faith will be. His Word dispels our doubts. Would you like to open your heart to God and by faith receive His power today? If you desire to enter into a new relationship of trust and confidence in God, you can ask Him to give you a trusting heart so that you can experience the health benefits of a living faith.

[1] In David N. Elkins, "Spirituality," available online at http://psychologytoday.com/articles/199909/spirituality.

[2] *Ibid.*

[3] *Ibid.*

[4] *Ibid.*

[5] *Ibid.*

[6] *Ibid.*

[7] Quoted by Sharon Jayson, "Power of a Super Attitude," *USA Today,* Oct.12, 2004, available at http://usatoday30.usatoday.com/news/health/2004-10-12-mind-body_x.htm.

Conclusion

HEALTH TO THE MAX

Hope is on the way: rejoice in it.

In April 2013 the city of St. Augustine, Florida, celebrated the 500th anniversary of the discovery of the Fountain of Youth. The Fountain of Youth is a legendary spring that supposedly restores the health and vigor of anyone who drinks or bathes in its bubbling waters. In the sixteenth century the story of healing waters became attached to the exploits of Spanish explorer Ponce de León, and St. Augustine is home of the Fountain of Youth Archaeological Park. The park is a tribute to the spot where tradition says Ponce de León first landed in America, although there's no clear documentation in his own writings that he discovered any such spring.

Nathaniel Hawthorne and other writers have used the metaphor of the Fountain of Youth in their tales. Even the Walt Disney Company in the United States got into the act by creating cartoons based on the legend.

Sagas of such a fountain have turned up worldwide for thousands of years, appearing in writings by Herodotus, the accounts of Alexander the Great, and the stories of Prester John, a legendary figure popular in Europe from the twelfth through the seventeenth centuries. Similar legends were also prominent among the Caribbean natives, who told tales of the healing powers of the waters in the mythical land of Bimini.

The problem with such fountains of youth, however, is that people who drink the "magical" water and bathe in its fountains still get old, they still get sick, and they still die. Although hundreds of thousands of tourists have visited St. Augustine's Fountain of Youth throughout the years, their health hasn't improved much.

Millions of people worldwide also pursue their own "fountains" of eternal youth. Whether it's a plant-based natural diet, a rigorous exercise regime, positive thinking, or some wonder cream to reduce wrinkles, we all long to discover something that will extend our lives and perpetuate our youthful exuberance. Within each one of us is a divinely placed desire to live a long, healthy, happy life. Obviously we want the most abundant life possible, and the principles discussed in this book will help us to live life to the full and likely to extend it, but they will not enable us to live forever.

Recent research into lifestyle issues has strongly confirmed that adhering to some basic principles of health can lengthen our lives by seven years or more—but how significant is that when viewed in the light of human history?

This leads us to one of life's most important questions: Is there a fountain of eternal youth whose waters really will satisfy our inner longing for eternity? Deep within our hearts we crave a remedy to the sickness, suffering, and sorrow that stalk our land. We want a solution for disease, disaster, and death. So let us finish this book with a fascinating journey of discovery to the *true* fountain of eternal youth.

The Real Fountain of Youth

Two thousand years ago on a sweltering summer afternoon in Palestine, Jesus met a brokenhearted woman longing for something more in her life but desperately afraid to admit it. The hollow relationships she had had with multiple men only reinforced her poor self-image. Seeking someone to care for her as a person, she hoped beyond hope to fill the emptiness in her soul. Then she met Jesus. Different than any other man she had ever encountered, He showed her respect, listened carefully to her story, and responded kindly. He seemed to know everything about her before she revealed it, but still accepted her with a noncondemning attitude.

As the conversation unfolded, the Samaritan woman realized that Jesus was the Messiah. In a remarkable moment as they sat on the side of Jacob's Well, He said: "Whoever drinks of this water will thirst again, but whoever drinks of the water that I shall give him will never thirst. But the water that I shall give him will become in him a fountain of water springing up into everlasting life" (John

4:13, 14, NKJV). The divine Christ offered the woman a drink from the true fountain of youth.

Jesus satisfies. He cleanses. And He provides eternal life. Scores of substitutes and counterfeits exist, but there is only one true Messiah. Only one Person can really satisfy the deepest needs of the human heart and provide eternal life.

Speaking to the Jewish leaders and multitudes locked in religious ritual, Jesus invited them: "If anyone thirsts, let him come to Me and drink. He who believes in Me as the scripture has said, out of his heart shall flow rivers of living water" (John 7:37, 38, NKJV). By coming to Jesus, we receive the gift of eternal life. Heaven begins in our hearts now. There springs up a new peace, a new power for daily living, and a new hope for the future.

For the Bible-believing Christian, death is not a long night without a morning. Nor is it a dark hole in the ground or a tunnel with no light at the end of it. Jesus stated it succinctly: "Let not your heart be troubled; you believe in God, believe also in Me. In My Father's house are many mansions; if it were not so, I would have told you. I go to prepare a place for you. And if I go and prepare a place for you, I will come again and receive you to Myself; that where I am, there you may be also" (John 14:1-3, NKJV).

Our Lord has an eternal answer to the problem of sickness and suffering, as well as our anxieties about aging. One day Jesus will come again. Then He will re-create our planet, so tainted with sin and suffering, to be like the Garden of Eden. He will make new heavens and a new earth (2 Peter 3:13). Cancer and heart disease will be no more. The doors of every emergency room will close forever, and all hospitals will go out of business. They will have no diseases to treat and no malignancies to cure.

John the revelator describes the healing river, the true fountain of youth: "And he showed me a pure river of water of life, clear as crystal, proceeding from the throne of God and the Lamb. In the middle of its street, and on either side of the river, was the tree of life, which bore twelve fruits, each tree yielding its fruit every month. The leaves of the tree were for the healing of the nations" (Revelation 22:1-3, NKJV). Talk about the fountain of youth—this is it! The book of Revelation pictures Eden restored. It depicts a new world with happy, healthy, and holy beings. This new world will fulfill our heart's longings, meet our deepest needs, satisfy our soul's hunger, and quench our inner thirst. Bathed in His loving presence, we will live in an atmosphere of love with the God who is love.

Heaven Is a Real Place

Heaven is a real place for real people. It's not some ethereal, make-believe world of disembodied spirits. Jesus declared, "Blessed are the meek, for they shall inherit the earth" (Matthew 5:5, NKJV). Peter adds, "Nevertheless we, according to His promise, look for a new heavens and a new earth in which righteousness dwells" (2 Peter 3:13, NKJV). Looking down the ages with prophetic insight, the apostle John testifies, "Now I saw a new heaven and a new earth, for the first heaven and the first earth had passed away" (Revelation 21:1, NKJV).

Imagine such a scene: living green carpets the earth's surface. Flowers in an infinite array of colors dot the landscape. Crystal-clear brooks wind their way through the green fields. The birds sing their happy songs. Animals of all shapes and sizes frolic in the sunlight. Joy and peace fill the land. Life and love flow from the heart of God, and all the new Eden's inhabitants rejoice in the atmosphere of the divine presence.

In the light of God's all-embracing love and forgiveness, fractured relationships have now healed. All tension is gone. Barriers no longer exist between people as harmony and unity replace estrangement and separation. Trust, belonging, and acceptance banish suspicion, conflict, and rejection.

The prophet Isaiah states it beautifully: "They shall not hurt nor destroy in all My holy mountain, for the earth shall be full of the knowledge of the Lord as the waters cover the sea" (Isaiah 11:9, NKJV). All our hurt and pain will be totally, completely, fully healed. We will be physically, mentally, emotionally, and spiritually whole.

Sin has separated us from God. Alienated from Him, we're disconnected from the source of total health. As a result, we endure anxiety and fear, sickness and disease, guilt and condemnation, bitterness and anger. But by accepting Jesus' love, receiving His grace, and embracing His power, we can not only live abundant lives here and now, but can reside with Him for eternity.

Following the principles the Lord has written on every nerve and tissue of our bodies, we can experience life at its best in a broken world, but the lingering effects of sin still remain. There are hereditary and environmental factors we cannot control. Sickness is still present. Although we may follow the Creator's laws of health faithfully, we still age. Death still lurks around the corner. But the vibrant hope that encourages all believers is that a better day will come. In his letter to Titus, the apostle Paul calls it the "blessed hope" (Titus 2:13). The hope of the return of Jesus and the glories of eternity lift our spirits, encourage our hearts, and inspire our lives.

In the United States a widely respected Michigan man known as "Uncle Johnson" died at 120 years of age. Perhaps one could credit his advanced years, at least in part, to the cheerful outlook that characterized his life. One day while at work in his garden during his later years, for example, he was singing songs of praise to God. His pastor, who was passing by, looked over the fence and said, "Uncle Johnson, you seem very happy today."

"Yes," the old man answered. "I was just thinking."

"Thinking about what?"

"Just that if the crumbs of joy that fall from the Master's table in this world are so good, what will the great loaf in glory be like! I tell you, sir, there will be enough for everyone, and some to spare up there."

The old man was right. The joy we experience here is just a faint reflection of the overwhelming one we will have in the light of God's amazing glory. The promise of "new heavens and a new earth" gives us the courage to face whatever life throws at us today and whatever challenges we're confronted with tomorrow.

The apostle Paul inspired the church at Corinth with these incredible words: "Behold, I tell you a mystery: We shall not all sleep, but we shall all be changed—in a moment, in the twinkling of an eye, at the last trumpet. For the trumpet will sound, and the dead will be raised incorruptible, and we shall be changed. For this corruptible must put on incorruption and this mortal must put on immortality" (1 Corinthians 15:51-53, NKJV).

The word "mortal" simply means subject to deterioration, decay, disease, and death. The word "immortal," conversely, means not subject to those things. Based on the promises of our Lord Himself, He will return and transform our weak, disease-prone bodies into glorious immortal ones, and we shall never be sick again.

Beyond Our Wildest Dreams

The Bible is full of wonderful promises that God will fulfill His plan for our total well-being (see Isaiah 33:24; 35:5, 6). Then we shall build houses and inhabit them, plant vineyards and eat the fruit from them, and long enjoy the work of our hands (see Isaiah 65:21-23). With healthy new bodies filled with vitality and abounding with energy, we will live as we were created to do so in the beginning. We will find incredible satisfaction in utilizing our God-given creativity and expanding our minds to the fullest. As we explore the secrets of the universe, we will ever marvel at God's incredible goodness.

God will forever erase the emotional scars of the past. Childhood hurts will have healed. The crushing blows of life that suddenly thrust themselves upon us will be swallowed up in an ocean of Christ's grace. "[For] the ransomed of the Lord shall return, and come to Zion with singing, with everlasting joy upon their heads. They shall obtain joy and gladness, and sorrow and sighing shall flee away" (Isaiah 35:10, NKJV). In the presence of Christ we shall have joy everlasting.

Nothing must prevent you from missing this. By God's grace and power, you can choose the best total health today, prepare to see your Savior face to face in the earth made new, and experience unending happiness throughout all eternity.

CONTRIBUTORS
AND CONSULTANTS

Albert Reece
Physician

Allan Handysides
Physician

Benjamin Carson
Neurosurgeon

Clifford Goldstein
Writer

Delbert W. Baker
Theologian

Duane McBride
Sociologist

Fred Hardinge
Physician

Katia Reinert
Nurse

Mark A. Finley
Pastor

Gary Fraser
Researcher

Gary Hopkins
Researcher

Peter N. Landless
Physician

Neil Nedley
Physician

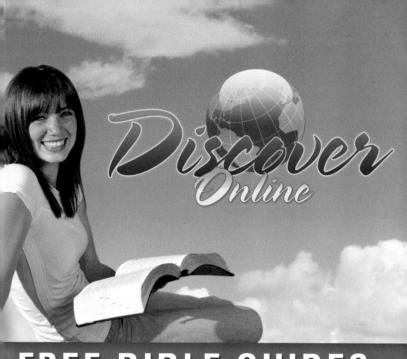

FREE BIBLE GUIDES

It's easy to learn more about the Bible!

Request: www.biblestudies.com/request

Write: Discover
P.O. Box 2525
Newbury Park, CA 91319

Call: 1-888-456-7933

Study Online: www.bibleschools.com

Offering **God's good news** for a better life
today and for eternity

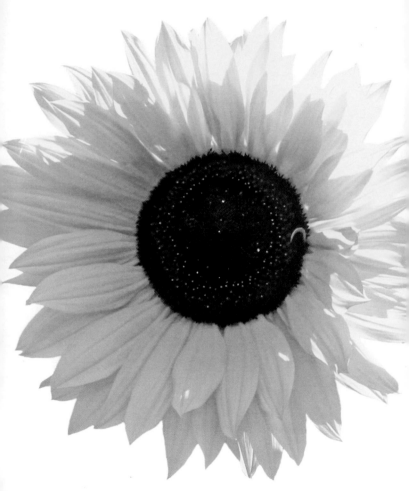

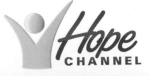 **Hope** CHANNEL

hopetv.org
Christian television programing about faith
health, relationships, and community